Fat Kid Got Fit

Bill in 1994 . . .   *. . . and Bill today*

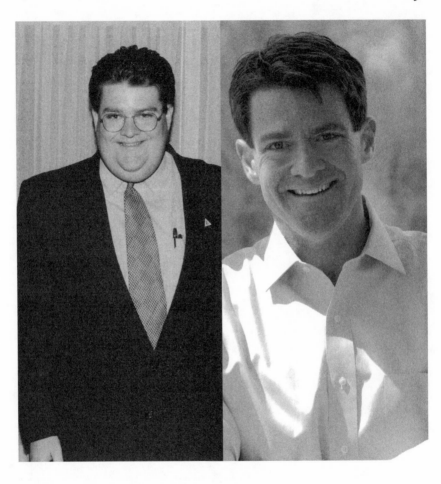

FAT KID
GOT FIT
And So Can You!

BILL BARONI
with
Damon DiMarco

with a foreword by
Dr. Howard Eisenson,
Executive Director of the Duke University Diet & Fitness Center

LYONS PRESS
Guilford, Connecticut
An imprint of Globe Pequot Press

Lyons Press is an imprint of Globe Pequot Press.

Text design: Sheryl P. Kober
Layout: Mary Ballachino
Project editor: Kristen Mellitt

Library of Congress Cataloging-in-Publication Data is available on file.

ISBN 978-0-7627-7047-2

Printed in the United States of America

10 9 8 7 6 5 4 3 2 1

To my mom, Geraldine Baroni,
whom I miss every day and
who I wish had seen her
Fat Kid Get Fit.

To my sister, Christine,
who showed me what being fit means
and how much I could miss someone.

To Dad and June,
who lived my weight loss with me.

CONTENTS

Contents

FOREWORD

BY DR. HOWARD EISENSON,

*Executive Director of the Duke University
Diet & Fitness Center*

In 1999 I accepted a position as Medical Director at the Duke Diet and Fitness Center (the DFC), a residential weight loss and lifestyle change program at Duke University, in Durham, North Carolina. At the time, I was not an expert in obesity treatment, nor did I have a particular passion for working with obesity as a medical condition. However, as a family physician in a typical office-based practice, I certainly had worked with many people for whom excess weight—and poor physical fitness—were major obstacles to good health. And, like most physicians, I felt frustrated that I had little to offer these people; in fact, I could count on the fingers of one hand the number of patients I had treated who had managed to achieve significant and lasting weight loss, or who had become regular exercisers and substantially boosted their level of physical fitness. The idea of working in a center where I would be part of a multidisciplinary team, where I would have the time and the resources to help motivated individuals accomplish real change, held great appeal. I felt then, as now, that surely one of the greatest goals of medicine must be to empower people to achieve optimal wellness—and I thought that the Duke Diet and Fitness Center could be a place where that would happen routinely.

Twelve years later, and now leading the center, I have learned a lot and am so grateful to have had the opportunity to be part of this special place. I have worked with thousands of patients, and despite many successes along the way I remain humbled by the fact that this is really challenging work. It is not enough for the treatment professionals to know their field, for the patients to be intelligent and highly motivated, for us to teach state-of-the-science behavior change skills and to coach people as they practice them. In short, lifestyle change is difficult. For so many of us, indeed for most of us, our biology and our modern environment make it very easy, perhaps even "normal," to eat too much and to exercise too little. As I say to our new patients in my introductory lecture each week, in a real sense we are proposing that they undertake a *life* change rather than a *lifestyle* change—a change that involves examining one's priorities and values, the choices we make about how and with whom we spend our time, our relationship to our work, how we organize our days, the "conversations" we have with ourselves, perhaps even where we live and who we live with.

It's a bigger deal than I realized, certainly bigger than most of my patients realize at first. Yet if we can make that critical decision to truly place a priority on our health, to recognize that there will inevitably be roadblocks along the way, to create strategies for dealing with those road-blocks, and to accept that ultimately the choice and the responsibility to change are ours, we can achieve success and the benefits can be amazing.

I wish I could say that Bill Baroni is our typical patient, that success like his is routinely achieved by the patients we serve. That's simply not the case. Bill is extraordinary and his success is remarkable. But I assure you that he is a real person, with genuine challenges in his own life. Like so many others he decided he wanted something better for himself. He wanted to be able to live life fully—with vigor and endurance, comfortable in body and in mind. But unlike many others, he realized that ultimately he was responsible for achieving the results he wanted. Others could provide support and encouragement, but no one else could make good choices for him—and no one could stop him. People often ask me what I think are the key factors predicting success in lifestyle change. Bill Baroni, and others like him, have taught me that real people, with real challenges, can achieve truly great success—so great in fact that many have proclaimed, "I got my life back." Nothing is more reward-ing for a doctor to hear. I have learned that success is most likely when the individual finally recognizes, "It's up to me." One's work may be very demanding, relationships may be stressful, time and money may be powerful constraints. But ultimately, the person who "gets their life back" refuses to be a victim any longer—he (or she) recognizes that lifestyle change is indeed within their power and that the regular practice of healthy habits can work for them.

Bill Baroni feels a genuine kinship with so many others who have suffered the pain—physical and emotional—of obesity and poor physical fitness. He is very generous in his praise of the Duke Diet and Fitness Center and of the important role the center played in helping him to realize his own potential for a full and rewarding life as a healthy and fit person. However, he recognizes that most people cannot afford the expense or the time to come to a place like the DFC, and this book is his generous gift to them. The ingredients for success are all here: Accept the fact that real and lasting improvement in your health requires that you adopt healthy habits for life—what we call "lifestyle change"; recognize that while a deep and lasting commitment is called for, perfection is not required—a host of practical real-world strategies make the task doable, one day at a time (with humor and empathy, Bill offers a wonderful collection of tips that has worked for him and can work for you too); and finally, identify a community of folks who appreciate what you are going through and will support your efforts, as you in turn support them.

Over the years of our association, Bill Baroni has taught me a lot and has truly been a source of inspiration. I sincerely hope that this honest, heartfelt account of his own journey to better health will inspire and help you as well. Throughout this book Bill tells us, "If I did it, you can too." He means it—and you can.

PART ONE:

FAT KID

I Almost Died in the Men's Room at the Meadowlands Racetrack

Everybody talks about *That Moment*. The one that changes your life forever. I guess this was mine.

In the summer of 1994, I was twenty-two years old and working as the driver and political aide-de-camp for Garabed "Chuck" Haytaian, speaker of the New Jersey State Assembly. Chuck was running for the United States Senate and he'd planned an ambitious campaign, one for which he and I often would spend fourteen, sixteen, eighteen hours a day driving all over the state of New Jersey, from speech to speech and lunch to lunch, from campaign event to campaign event. Sometimes we covered ten venues a day. It was a crazy schedule but a very exciting time.

I was finishing my history degree from George Washington University and I planned on going to law school. But then this job with Chuck came up, and how could I turn it down? I'd worked in politics since I was a teenager, and being a candidate's driver is one of the greatest jobs you can get. You get to see and experience all the details of a campaign. You get to see the political process in action, good and bad, and I hoped that, if Chuck won the election, I'd accompany him to Washington. But if he lost? Well, like I said. Law school was always waiting.

Running for office is a tough grind and we worked hard. Chuck and I were up and on the road at five o'clock nearly every morning. I drove him back and forth to events in a souped-up Ford Econoline van we called (you guessed it) the Chuck Wagon. Chuck lived in Hackettstown, which is way up in the northwest part of the state in Warren County, right on the Delaware River. I knew the days were going to be long (they turned out to be practically endless) and I didn't want to lump a commute on top of all the other hours I was logging. So I rented a small, windowless basement apartment in a neighborhood a few miles away from Chuck's house. It made my morning drive and evening commute much easier.

Each morning, I'd climb in the van and drive to Chuck's condo. Chuck would always be ready for breakfast so we'd head to a local bakery called Harpers to order some donuts and coffee. We'd spend a while getting caught up on the news of the day before we left Hackettstown. The donuts at Harpers were pretty outstanding, so sometimes I ordered two. Okay, sometimes three. What can I say? I was hungry. Chuck and I were working hard and our appetites were up. We told ourselves we needed a good breakfast to get ready for the long day ahead.

When we finished eating, we'd walk back out to the parking lot and climb back into the van. The Chuck Wagon's shock absorbers would groan a little in protest. At that point, I weighed over three hundred pounds. The driver's seat of the Ford Econoline van suffered the penalty of all those donuts.

Political campaigns often revolve around food. On a typical day, Chuck and I would hit two or three breakfasts followed by two or three lunches. Each time Chuck took the podium to address the crowd, I would stand off in a corner somewhere with a cell phone jammed in my ear, coordinating the next stop along the trail. Meanwhile, people pressed plates of food into our hands wherever we went, and we couldn't say no. Civic associations, the Kiwanis, the local Chamber of Commerce— they all went to great trouble to organize meetings where elected officials could meet their constituents. It would have been impolite not to eat the food they'd ordered. We appreciated their support, so we ate. Again. And again. And again. Sometimes six or seven times, and that was just during the day. We'd hit two or three dinners each evening on average, and each dinner served was a full course meal. After a long career in politics, Chuck knew how to moderate his eating. Me? Not so much.

When it comes to entrees, political dinners can sort of resemble the meals served in incarceration facilities. Typically, we'd get a plate of chicken or fish or sometimes beef (which was always prime rib). Once in a while, whoever was hosting the event really pulled out the stops and treated us to Italian-themed soirees, Indian cuisine, or—in Chuck's case—lots of Armenian delicacies. Chuck was one of the highest-elected Armenian-Americans in the nation, and the community rightly embraced him. For dessert, there was always fresh pastry, homemade cookies, and cake.

By the end of each day, Chuck and I were exhausted. We'd climb back into the Chuck Wagon, and I'd crank it up and aim it toward home. From there, I'd drive us back to north Jersey while Chuck sat reading the many reports that had been sent to us from our campaign headquarters over the mobile fax machine.

We usually got back to Hackettstown about ten o'clock at night, and we often went to the Hackettstown Diner where we took a booth, compared notes, and planned the next day's events. I'd order the roast turkey with gravy. Sometimes I shook things up a bit and ordered the meatball sandwich instead. Finish up. Call for the check. Pay it. Drop tip. Back outside to the parking lot. Into the Chuck Wagon. Start the engine. That was the routine. Most nights, I'd drop Chuck at his house around midnight, wiped out from the day's events.

Chuck would always end the night excited to be home with his amazing wife Joan, and upbeat about the campaign. He and I had grown close in the course of our work, and I admired his commitment. I thought that Chuck had a lot to offer public service.

Sometimes people would ask me if I would ever run for office—but then, very quickly, they'd say, "Nah. You're a great behind-the-scenes guy, right?" I used to hear this so often that I started to think so, too. Because that's what I'd taught myself to say, the role I'd cast myself in. Like I said, I'd always wanted a career in politics. But I was also fat, and I had it in my head that I couldn't get elected.

At any rate, I'd wave good-bye to Chuck each night and drive the Chuck Wagon back to my tiny, dark apartment in Hackettstown, but I didn't go directly home. Most nights I still felt hungry, or at least very empty inside (at this point in my life, I hadn't yet learned how to separate the two). So I'd steer the Chuck Wagon toward the main strip that ran through the center of town and I'd hit the late-night drive-throughs.

Back then Hackettstown had a Burger King right next to a McDonald's. I'd always hit the McDonald's first and order extra large fries plus a Coke. Why just fries and a Coke? Because, in my considerable experience, McDonald's sold superior french fries—thin, salty, perfectly fried–and a Coke was the perfect soft drink to wash all those french fries down.

But that was just the opening act. Once I'd hit the McDonald's, I would swing the Chuck Wagon back onto the strip, drive about fifteen feet or so, and pull into the Burger King drive-through. At Burger King, I ordered fried chicken sandwiches as well as the estimable bacon double cheeseburger. Because again, in my considerable experience, Burger King fried superior chickens. And they certainly made a superior bacon double cheeseburger.

With those great smelling bags at my side, I'd head home, where I'd sit in my windowless basement apartment and lay out all my purchases on my tiny table. But they didn't sit on the table for long because I'd practically inhale them. And soon—very soon—I began to feel full. Wonderfully, blissfully, gorgeously full. In practical terms, this meant I was numb enough from stuffing myself that I could fall into bed, grab a few hours' sleep, get up, and go back to work again. Day after day. And every night, I was able to fill the emptiness I felt with fast food. My depression, if that's what it was, would disappear for a while.

Until.

In mid-June, I drove Chuck east to the New Jersey Meadowlands just outside New York City. For those of you who aren't familiar with it, the Meadowlands is a massive sports complex whose buildings have changed a bit over the years. Back in 1994, the indoor stadium was called the Brendan Byrne Arena (today it's known as the Izod Center). There's also the famous Meadowlands Racetrack for horse racing—harness and thoroughbred. And of course there was Giants Stadium (which the Jets and the Giants both called home, but we won't get into that).

At any rate, Giants Stadium was slated to host the upcoming Group E round of the FIFA World Cup that year. Everyone was excited. Sports fans were happy. The media was everywhere. Businesses were gearing up to reap a windfall of profits. It was the perfect place for a candidate to show up and press the flesh. That's how Chuck and I found ourselves at the famous Pegasus restaurant on the penthouse floor of the Meadowlands Racetrack.

The Pegasus was incredible! The place had a sumptuous interior. Everything was done up in jockey couture—leather, dark woods, polished brass, and marble wherever you looked. While Chuck took a meeting with officials visiting from across the globe, I ambled away from the table and hit the relative quiet of the bar. It seemed like the perfect place to take out my cell phone and check messages. So that's what I did—or started to, anyway. Before I'd even gotten to voicemail, I was rudely interrupted by deep and shooting pains that hit my chest like a blow from a spear. I gasped and nearly dropped the phone and thought, *Whoa! Hold on there, wait just a sec! What the heck was that? We have a problem!*

The pains struck again, even harder. Then harder. Sort of like they were answering me. *This?* the pains seemed to be saying. *Why, this is a heart attack, Bill. You've heard about them—everyone has—and this is what they feel like!*

I panicked. I didn't know what to do, so I rushed to the door of the men's room, yanked it open, and stumbled inside.

Thank God the bathroom was empty. The pains struck again and I thought, *I'm dying! This is it, I'm dying, I'm dying at the Pegasus restaurant. Good Lord, here I go . . .*

Barreling straight to the sink, I turned on the cold water tap full blast and shoveled the water onto my face. I was scared. No, that's not exactly right. I was absolutely *terrified*. I couldn't believe what was happening.

My God, I thought. *I'm twenty-two years old and I thought I'd have so much time. But here I am having a heart attack in a men's room out at the Meadowlands and this awful Muzak keeps playing over and over and I hate it and I'm dying. This is what dying feels like. It's worse than elevator music . . .*

It was not a very good moment for me.

The pains hit again and I stood there, clutching the lip of the marble sink, gasping like I'd just run a mile (it was really more like fifty feet . . . well, okay, maybe forty). *Breathe*, I told myself. *Just breathe.* I remember lifting my head and staring into the mirror, which confused me. It took me a second to recognize what I was seeing. I didn't understand why there was a bright pink soccer ball where my head should be. Then the soccer ball blinked and I remember nearly fainting. *Wait a minute!* I thought. *That's* me! *That's my* face! *I'm fat, and I'm dying because I'm so heavy.*

So I stood there with one hand clutching my chest. I waited to die . . . but it didn't happen. The pains gave a tweak, then a half-hearted twinge, and then they gave up and began to subside. I can't even say I felt any relief. Just this incredible, lingering shock that seemed to stop the world on its axis, leaving everything strange and still, but tilted at odd angles. It was the way it feels right after you've survived an auto accident (which I had done) or a fall down the stairs.

I took a few minutes to gather myself and staggered back out to the dining room. Chuck was just getting ready to go; he was shaking hands all around. I joined him in saying good-bye to all and we left the Pegasus.

As we walked toward the car, I remember very clearly thinking, *I'm the fat kid who almost died. Right over there in the men's room.*

I thought of the face that I'd seen in the mirror and that's when I realized I had to change. I'd been given a second chance at life. But would I take it? That was the question. Really, that's *always* the question.

My Moment had arrived.

I Think I Know Why You're Here

Why did you pick up this book? Why are you reading these words right now? I think I know. It's not that hard to figure out. I chose the title to resonate with a certain group of folks—people, like me, whose lives have been defined by our size. People who are fat. Maybe you're just a few pounds overweight. Maybe you're like I was: a lot of pounds overweight. Either way, we'll use the same term. We're all fat, and we want to get fit.

But it's not so easy, is it? Trust me, I know. I've been there. It's tough. Or, no—I'm sorry, I take that back. Tough is just the beginning. Getting fit is one of the hardest challenges life can throw at you. Sometimes you try and you try and you try but it just doesn't seem to work. Which makes you lose faith. Which makes you lose hope. Which makes you give up. Which makes life seem awful. I get it. I've been there. I know.

Maybe you're in a bad spot right now. Maybe you're frustrated. Maybe you're scared. Maybe you've simply given up hope, or maybe you know someone who has (maybe you picked up this book for them).

Am I right?

Look, if I'm wrong, I apologize. Put this book down and walk away. I wish you well on your journey. But if I'm right, then I think we should talk. Because you're the person I wrote this book for. You and me and people like us. You're not alone. Not anymore.

If I'm right about who I think you are, you're looking at the road ahead, and you think it's too far to walk. You're looking at your body and wondering how you could ever possibly lose that weight. Maybe it's always been there, like a reassuring friend. Maybe you've tried to lose it before and you've failed. Maybe you think that you'll try again and fail a second time. Or a third. Or a fourth. A fifth or a sixth. Maybe a part of you has started to think that being fit—being "normal" (whatever that means) or alive—is only for other people. Not you.

So how can a guy like *me* help *you*? Because I made my journey from fat to fit, and I did it without bariatric surgery. Without drugs. Without trendy exercise equipment. Expensive products. The latest diet craze. Sadly, the list of fakirs and false prophets in this game of getting fit goes on and on and on.

I lost my weight using common sense. And if I can do it, so can you.

The Doctor Will NOT See You Now

There's something I need to get straight right off the bat. Actually, a couple of things. For starters:

- *I am not a medical doctor*—I have deep respect for those folks who are. I cannot and will not dispense medical advice. Couple everything I say in this book with your doctor's advice and counsel.

- *I am not a guru*—frankly, I distrust gurus. I have a profession outside of this field. Which means that I'm probably just like you, someone whose job demands much of his time. Who maintains other interests.

- *I don't hold degrees in nutrition, body mechanics, or exercise*— everything that I've learned so far has come through my own experience as a fat person getting fit. So that's the perspective I'll talk to you from. The place that I'm writing from.

Apart from this book, I'm not trying to sell you anything. I don't take endorsements from exercise products or health clubs or anything like that. I don't want you to watch my reality TV show. I don't even *have* a reality TV show.

So who am I? Like I said: I'm just a guy who lost a lot of weight and found a way to keep it off. How did I do it? I used common sense tips. Some dedication. Some education. An amazing support network. And, okay, I think I can give myself this: a deep and lasting commitment. In other words, I wouldn't give up. I told myself I deserved to be fit, and then I followed through. I was never going back to that men's room. Never ever again.

But just so I'm clear: I did not spend a fortune. I didn't apprentice myself to some mystic who taught me ancient weight-loss secrets. I don't work out for three hours a day. I love my life. I love staying fit. I'm having a great time. So can you. I truly believe that everyone deserves to live the life they envision for themselves, and that's why I'd like to share my findings with you. I want to help you to get where you want to be: a healthier, happier, fitter you.

If this sounds like something you're interested in, fantastic. Keep reading. I think we'll have lots to discuss. But the first thing I want to acquaint you with is a set of pretty scary facts.

Obesity Is a National Health Crisis

You've heard it on the TV news and read about it in the papers. Nowadays it seems like every major print magazine and television program has told the same story time and again: American waistlines have started to bulge, and they're showing no signs of stopping.

In fact, as I write this book, the latest studies indicate that *more than two-thirds of American adults are overweight.* That's right, I said over two-thirds. The same studies say that *over one-third of adult Americans are clinically obese.*[1] Let's pause here and figure out what that means.

If you really wanted to, you could find out whether you're technically overweight or obese by calculating your body mass index (BMI). Your BMI is a number. Think of it as a score that ranges from 18 and under to 35 and over. Your BMI score indicates how much body fat you carry based on normal heights and weights for adult men and women. Typically, a person is considered overweight if their BMI falls between 25 and 29.9. A BMI over 30 indicates obesity. Calculating your BMI is easy. Just visit a website set up by the U.S. Department of Health and Human Services at www.nhlbisupport.com/bmi.

But remember this: Your BMI score isn't some absolute. For instance, people who are very muscular will often have a high BMI, but it doesn't mean that they're overweight. Their bodies are heavier than most, more dense, but that's with muscle, not fat. And BMI doesn't take into consideration, for example, elderly people who've lost a lot of muscle tissue but carry a lot of fat instead. So I'm telling you: Don't get hung up on these numbers. If you check out your BMI at all, I recommend using it as a benchmark, and that's it.

And really, your BMI is irrelevant from the most important point of view. It doesn't matter what technical classification you fall into. *I* knew I was fat back then. *You* know you're carrying too much weight now. You know it better than anyone. You can feel the weight dragging you down every day, and maybe it's making your life pretty hard. Maybe it's making you miserable. Maybe you have those moments like I did, moments when you're alone in the basement, depressed and eating fast food. To which I say that's a good first step. Knowing that you're miserable and wanting to feel better each day is all the motivation you need to start losing weight and keep it off. Not just for a few weeks, by the way, or a few months, or even a year or two. I mean getting the weight off and keeping it off for good. For the rest of your life.

Who cares if you're clinically overweight as opposed to clinically obese? Either condition puts you at risk to develop some really awful health problems, the most common of which include:

- type 2 diabetes

- hypertension and high LDL (or "bad" cholesterol, which often leads to heart disease and strokes)

- certain forms of cancer, notably breast, kidney, colorectal, and endometrial cancer

- nonalcoholic fatty liver disease

- gallbladder disease

- sleep apnea and other breathing problems

- osteoarthritis, in which your cartilage, bones, and joints start to degenerate as they're literally crushed under the weight of your body

- for women, menstrual irregularities and complications during pregnancy[2]

Wow. None of that sounds really good, am I right? And the situation's bound to get worse. In fact, I'm willing to bet that the average American's weight has *increased*. Scales are tipping. Waistlines have grown. Complications from being fat have risen into the stratosphere. And why not? *Obesity has reached epidemic proportions by the clinical definition of the word.* In other words, in battling our weights, modern Americans face a disease that's our generation's equivalent of polio, smallpox, and tuberculosis rolled into one. And the costs incurred by battling this epidemic are staggering. For instance, consider that:

- The United States experienced a 76 percent increase in adult onset type 2 diabetes for people in their thirties since 1990 (as a disease, type 2 diabetes is perfectly preventable given proper diet, nutrition, and exercise).[3]

- Within the same short period, we've seen a 70 percent rise in cardiovascular diseases related to obesity.

- In 2001, the Centers for Disease Control (CDC) and several independent assessors agreed that *the economic toll attributable to obesity in the United States hit a staggering $75 billion that year.* In 2008, the CDC revised its figures saying that costs has risen to $147 billion.[4] What do you think the costs are *now*? How high do you think they have climbed? Read the next bullet point.

- One study published in December 2010 by the Society of Actuaries pegged the revised economic toll as being *$270 billion per year!* Think about that for a moment. From $75 billion in 2001 to $270 billion in 2010 . . . that's nearly a fourfold cost increase in less than a decade! The authors of the Society of Actuaries' study say that close to half this money goes to excess medical care. Other allocations include loss of national productivity due to increased mortality and economic loss of productivity due to workers' disability. Furthermore, the authors note that, of these sums, approximately one-third are derived from persons being overweight, while closer to two-thirds are actually caused by obesity.[5]

Also according to the CDC :

- Obese children carry an increased risk of developing a wide variety of physical and psychological disorders.
- Overweight adolescents have a 70 percent chance of becoming overweight or obese adults.
- Obese adults have a 50 to 100 percent increased risk of premature death from all causes. Think about what that means: a 100 percent chance. Those aren't very good odds.

Given all this, it probably comes as no surprise that:

- Various sources estimate that one-quarter of the American population eats fast food at least once every day.
- The average child ages 8 to 18 will spend 13 to 14 hours a week playing video games.
- According to the Pentagon, the number of U.S. troops diagnosed as overweight or obese has doubled since the start of the War in Iraq.[6]
- Nearly one-third of American children and teens ages 2 through 19 are clinically overweight or obese.[7]
- In the past 40 years, instances of being considered clinically overweight or obese have more than quadrupled among children ages 6 through 11, and more than tripled among adolescents ages 12 through 19.[8]
- The direct costs stemming from childhood obesity alone (this number includes such sub-brackets as prescription drugs, outpatient costs, and emergency room treatments) is a staggering $14.1 billion. Obesity-related illnesses cost the Medicare system $19.7 billion in 2008. In the same year, Medicaid paid out $8 billion for the same types of illness while private insurance plans paid $49 billion.[9]

I've listed a bunch of statistics and I hope they got your attention. But right about now, you're probably thinking, *So what? Statistics won't give me what I want. Statistics won't make me fit.*

Fair enough. I understand your frustration. Remember, I've been there, too. You want to move forward, but you don't know how, so you're chomping at the bit. In fact, if you're anything like I was before I lost my weight, you're probably really frustrated with one thing in particular. I remember it like this: I remember being fat and wondering . . .

Why Are All These Skinny People Shouting at Me!?!

When I was heavy, it seemed like the world was chock full of thin people telling me I should lose weight. Work harder, they said. Run faster. Eat less. Think this. Do that. Try so-and-so's product.

These thin people were plastered across every TV screen, smiling and hawking abdominal crunchers and cardio machines and kickboxing videos. I saw them in commercials for the low-fat menu at national chain family restaurants. They leered at me from the covers of books that hyped the latest "science" of weight loss. The chocolate diet! The cabbage diet! And many, many more.

Thin people were everywhere, flashing their sculpted six-pack abs and flexing their muscles and saying things like, "Getting in shape is as easy as watching my video! Buy it now!!"

I never listened to any of them. Sure, they were trying to get my attention, but just the opposite happened. I came to think, *Well, what do you know?* I didn't want to hear a thin person telling me I should exercise. Whenever I heard a thin person talking about exercise, I'd think:

Yeah, yeah, lady. Whatever you say. I get it. You're a size zero. Congratulations.

OR

Whoop-dee-doo, look who won the genetic lottery. Stop rubbing it in my face and get out of my way. I'm hungry and it's time for lunch . . .

OR

Sure, man, I see you're a thirty-inch waist with a fifty-inch chest, I get it. But look at me, will you? JUST LOOK AT ME! I can NEVER be like you!!

Well. I'm not going to talk to you like a thin person telling you you're fat. Thin people can't understand what we go through. They don't really speak the same language. It's like Thin People are from Mars and Fat People (like me) are from . . . reality.

I'm going to talk to you as someone who found a way to get thin. Because that's what I am and that's what I did. And so can you. I've lived through my obesity nightmare. I found a way out. And so can you.

Maybe you don't believe that. Maybe you're thinking, *I've always been heavy and heavy is what I will* always *be.* You know what? I used to think that way, too. I didn't just wake up fat one day—I'd been heavy all my life . . . until I decided I had to change. And then I went looking for answers that worked. And then I applied those answers. I found a way to make change stick. And yes, I have to say this again. Not for a month and not for a year. I'm making my change stick for good. And so can you.

You don't have to spend a small fortune. You don't have to starve yourself. You don't have to go home, pull open your refrigerator door, and throw out all your favorite foods. Here's the secret: You just have to start *thinking* differently. You just have to change your *lifestyle* a bit to include a few common sense tips. You have to create new habits. Start doing that and I'll bet you'll be shocked. You can lose weight, feel healthier, and gain more energy and confidence almost immediately. You can start becoming the person you've always wanted to be. Right now.

I just mentioned a word we're going to find ourselves using a lot—*lifestyle.* We're going to figure out what it really means, and how it's the key to keeping you fit. But before we get into that, I want you to know exactly where I'm coming from. I want you to know how hopeless my battle with weight always seemed, how growing up as a fat kid made me *feel.* Because maybe you've been there. Maybe you get it. And maybe you need to see that you're not alone.

Let me take a moment to tell you about . . .

The Perils of Being Fat and Young

I remember one time when I was talking to a friend, and I was saying (as I just said to you) that being overweight is an American epidemic. This friend replied:

> *Bill, you're wrong. You say that being overweight is a deadly disease, but you know what? Being overweight is worse than contracting a deadly disease. Because being heavy carries a different stigma. People are usually sympathetic when they find out you have an illness. But no one's sympathetic when you're heavy. They think you lack willpower, character, courage.*

So true! This friend of mine was right. He'd hit the nail right on the head, in fact, at least from my experience.

When I was overweight, that's exactly the kind of discrimination I faced from lots of people who weren't battling their weight. Most of them never openly stated their contempt. Polite society prefers that we hide such prejudices. But it was always there in the way they looked at me. In the subtle asides they used to make, or the things they *didn't* say (which often could be just as painful, maybe even more so).

I'll state this very simply: The shame invoked by being heavy can be crippling. Lots of times people don't know how to deal with it. They feel as though they can't turn to anyone for help or sympathy—not their family or friends. They feel like no one's willing to lend them a supportive ear. This can make you feel isolated. Terribly, awfully alone. And the contempt society often heaps upon heavy people is remarkably hypocritical.

Somehow it's acceptable to mock fat people. But how would we react if we saw that same scathing contempt aimed at cancer patients, or heart disease patients? I think you know the answer to that. I think you know how rightfully detestable society would find such behavior. And yet fat people face this kind of discrimination every day of their lives, and no one says a word about it. If anything, some people contribute eagerly.

The shame I felt about my weight led me to pull some interesting tricks. For instance, here's a very strong memory I have. At some point—I might have been ten or eleven—my weight had clearly become an issue, so my parents started weighing me at home using a bathroom scale. But I figured out that you could rig the mechanism. The scale had a little wheel that you could play with to move the dial backwards, so that's what I did. I set the scale so the weight began not at *zero* but *negative 20*. My parents didn't catch on until they took me to see my pediatrician, Dr. John Morgan.

I went to see Dr. Morgan every year for my checkup. I remember he was always very kind to me, and of course as part of my appointment, he'd measure my height and weight. This presented a problem, of course, since there was no way I could creep into Dr. Morgan's office ahead of time and preset his scale (though I thought about it a lot, and wished I could do it with all my heart).

Well. I remember the numbers came in that year and my parents were shocked. They thought I weighed X. Now I suddenly weighed X + 20. I was caught. Mom and dad figured out what I'd been doing pretty quick, and my oh my were they angry!

Looking back, I can totally understand the awful situation I'd put them in. Their reaction arose from their deep concern. Clearly, their son was heavy, but worse: He was getting even heavier. As if it wasn't obvious to the naked eye, Dr. Morgan's chart was always there to lend official confirmation. You know the chart I'm talking about: The one that shows the normal height and weight for a kid as he grows. My height was always in line, of course—that wasn't the issue at all. But as far as my weight? Well . . . you know the phrase "off the charts"? Let's just say that I know where it comes from.

Imagine my parents' dismay at all this. Remember, this was during the late 1970s or early '80s. Back then, no one talked about childhood obesity, or any kind of weight issues. In fact, a lot of talk about health was muted. I knew that my mom had been diagnosed with adult onset diabetes, which she controlled by taking Diabenese pills. My sister, Christine, and I had been adopted from different families. Our biological histories were always a big open question mark. But imagine my parents' confusion. Dad was thin and mom was thin and so was Christine. What difference did having different biological histories make? Weren't we all eating the same exact food? When Mom made pot roast for dinner, we all had pot roast. When mom made hot dogs, we all had hot dogs. But I was fat and they were not. So what was going on?

People rarely called me fat. If anything, they avoided that term as though it was a disease in itself. Early on, they told me that I had a little "baby fat." A few years later, they called me "husky." Then they started to use the word "stocky." Finally, they called me "big-boned," and that one struck me as really weird.

Big-boned? I thought. *That's ridiculous. Elephants are big-boned. So are hippopotami and Tyrannosaurus Rexes. Why don't we cut to the chase, okay? I'm fat. Do you hear me? I'm fat!*

Dr. Morgan would tell me I had to eat healthier, had to exercise. He took great pains to outline these issues, which made an impact on me. For a while. After appointments for annual checkups, I'd feel really bad, go home, close the door to my room, and do sit-ups. But that never lasted. Sit-ups aren't fun. They also never seemed to work. I'd stop the sit-ups a few days later and fall back into my normal routine (or lack thereof, more appropriately). Which meant that I remained fat.

And because I was fat, life was horrible. These days, I tell people that I never had any friends growing up. They smile and nod and say, "Sure, okay." I guess they think I'm exaggerating, but I'm not. I had no friends for years. I was the last kid picked (if I got picked at all) for every team in every game I ever played.

The fact is, many thin kids don't like having fat kids around. This isn't just my opinion, by the way, there's a famous study that proves it (we'll get to that later on). So I mostly hung out with adults. I learned pretty fast that grown-ups aren't so quick to discriminate against a kid's weight, especially if the fat kid in question is somewhat intelligent, laughs a lot, and acts like a perfect little adult, which of course I did. Frankly, it's one of the reasons I got interested in politics.

When I was fourteen, I volunteered at the office of my local congressman, Chris Smith. The congressman and his staff didn't care that I was fat. I could have been an alien from another planet, so long as I could lick envelopes and make a lot of phone calls. They cared if I could show up on time at campaign events and functions. They cared if I was willing to do the grunt work of politics, the stuff that no one else wanted to do. I was, so we got along fine. In many ways, the folks in Chris's campaign office were some of my first real friends. They were a caring, supportive family of people who welcomed me with open arms. This was the team behind Chris Smith, one of the country's leading advocates for human rights. To them, human rights seemed to include fat kids.

So my life with adults was going well, but my life with my peers was awful. Sometimes it was excruciating, like at that terrible point in each school year when we covered gymnastics in phys ed class. It still hurts whenever I think about it. The teachers would haul out the pommel horse and blow their whistles and tell everyone to line up.

Come on, I thought. *You can't be serious. Really? I mean, really?!?* Unfortunately, the gym teacher was serious, and to hell with Isaac Newton, right? Apparently, our gym teacher thought that the laws of physics were *made* to be broken. All I had to do was run right up to that springboard, jump, and I'd end up over the pommel horse (with perhaps the aid of a hot air balloon as well as a heavy-lift harbor crane). And once I'd vaulted the pommel horse, I'd flap my arms and fly away. Who says gravity always wins? Who doesn't believe in miracles?

And while we're at it, who can forget the great rope climb? Or the balance beam? *Balance?* Please. Being a fat kid in high-school gym class felt like having your back to the wall with a blindfold in front of a firing squad. It went beyond embarrassment. It was absolutely crippling. But I smiled. I joked. I deflected. Demurred. I did what I'd always done. I protected the sensitive man inside from all those barbs and acrid jests. I protected the man that no one could see, the one who had hidden himself so well that even I sometimes suspected he'd never existed at all.

Then one day our gym teacher took us running in the park across the street from the school. Well, that was the plan anyway. I couldn't run. I mean, come on . . . I got winded walking up one flight of stairs. Running? As in a mile or so? That was a joke, a physical impossibility. I knew it. So did everyone else. But that wasn't the worst part. Oh no. Not by far. The worst part was passing in front of the teacher and overhearing her tell other students, "Oh, that's okay if he walks. He *can't* run."

Because I'm fat, I thought. As I write this, I still feel the pain of that moment.

I remember another incident that happened in high school. A day or two after getting elected president of my junior class, I was riding my bike to the house of a friend, where we were going to study for final exams. Riding my bike wasn't unusual—I did it all the time. But this time on my way back home, I tried to cross the road and—WHAM!—a car smacked into me. The bike went flying and I went flying. We both landed on the pavement. I was bleeding and really hurt.

It was a pretty bad accident, but also a fortunate one. I can say that last part without hesitation because the local hospital was less than a hundred yards away. Also, an ambulance happened to be pulling out of the parking lot at the precise moment I got hit by the car. The paramedics saw what happened and raced right over to help me.

But at that point, I guess my luck ran out because, from there on in, the whole ordeal started to look like a sitcom. The paramedics had to wiggle a backboard under me so they could pick it up and slide me into the ambulance. They got me onto the board okay, but picking me up? Well, that was another story. Remember: These were paramedics, tough folks used to working hard. They sweated. They grunted. They used their legs and kept their backs straight and strained for all they were worth. But they still had a tough time lifting me. Why? You know why. I was fat.

I very clearly remember one of them saying, "Well! He's a really big boy!"

That comment hurt me a whole lot more than getting hit by the car. It was the way he said it. I'll never forget that—like an indictment, but worse than that, one that was based on incontrovertible evidence. I was guilty and I knew it.

You know how paramedics ask you questions when they're busy loading you into the back of an ambulance? They do that to keep you conscious, by the way, but also to make sure you're still rational, thinking clearly, in charge of your faculties. Well. They asked me my name, and I told them. "Bill." They asked me where I lived, and I told them that, too. Then they asked me if there was someone at home they should call. I told them my phone number and asked them to please call my mom. Then they asked me how old I was. I told them I was sixteen.

The look on both their faces. They were stunned, I tell you. Just stunned.

"Huh," said one, and he shot a look at the other. Then both of them looked at the bulk of my body, the massive cake of jiggling flesh they'd somehow managed to heave and shove and muscle into the back of the ambulance.

"Sixteen, huh?" the other one said. And then a short, flat: "Wow."

That was all they needed to say. I got the point, of course.

You'd think that an episode like that would inspire a fat kid to change his ways. Not so! I had to endure *another* collision—this next one also involved a car, and nearly turned out to be fatal. The kicker? I still didn't get the hint. I still wasn't willing to change.

The summer after my junior year in high school, I was hanging out with some friends I'd met at Boys State, a youth-in-government program the American Legion sponsors. A few of us drove down to the famous beach town of Wildwood on the southeast New Jersey coast. We were having such a fantastic time that somebody said we should pull an all-nighter and take a road trip further south to Washington, D.C. We didn't have a place to stay and we didn't have a reason to go. We just figured it would be fun to do. Ah, youth.

We all piled into my car—a dark blue 1981 Chevy Citation. We drove down the New Jersey Turnpike, over the Delaware Memorial Bridge, and made our way into Maryland. It was early morning, just before dawn. We'd been up all night. I was wiped out from driving so we stopped for a quick nap and I fell asleep in the backseat. One of my friends took the wheel and I was still snoozing in the backseat when the accident happened on I-95, somewhere just outside of Baltimore.

I woke up while our car was careening across traffic, and then it was run over by a truck. I remember the EMTs rushing in. They eventually pulled me out of the wreckage. They put me on a stretcher, then dropped me. Why? Because I was heavy.

I also remember when the MedEvac helicopter touched down on the roof of the University of Maryland at Baltimore's Shock/Trauma Hospital Center. How the paramedics grunted and heaved. How sweat rolled down their faces. They struggled to pull me out of the aircraft, onto the roof, and across the pad to get me to the ER. Grunting and heaving and sweating the same way the paramedics had the first time I'd been hit by a car. Only this time, I'd gotten fatter still. By then, I weighed about 275 pounds.

A frightening situation? Yes. Embarrassing? You bet, and potentially lethal, too. By that summer, I had gotten so big that the doctors had a tough time inspecting my body for damage. They knew that I howled in pain whenever someone touched my right leg. But that was all they could diagnose. My folds were hiding a lot from their eyes and made it hard for them to do their jobs. They thought I might have broken my neck or pelvis or fractured my spine. Frankly, nothing they said was great fun, but you know what? I wasn't frightened.

There! I've said it! You know what I really felt? Relief. One thought kept running around in my mind as those EMTs picked up my fat form and shouldered it clear across the big roof, then down to the ER and surgery. One thought and one thought only, which was: *Thank God! No swimming in gym class this year! I won't have to put on a bathing suit and wear it in front of everyone else! No gymnastics! No pommel horse!*

That was my biggest concern, of course, because everyone used to laugh at me. Did the laughter hurt? Oh yes. But the worst part of all was when the hurt stopped and numbness set in. The worst part was when I accepted the wounds, the constant snickers, the outright derision . . . and then the looks that followed—or didn't. The *didn't* part could be lethal, you know.

Fat people often get overlooked. People would rather not see them. As far as most of the world is concerned, it's better to simply pretend we're not there, to write us off like we don't exist.

And all the while, I wanted to change—not for anyone else's sake, but for mine. I wanted some help. I just wanted to start living again, but I didn't know how—where to start or who to ask. I felt powerless. Stupid. Locked in a box. Sad and angry at once.

The Damage Done by Addiction

I have the utmost respect for people who battle addiction to drugs and alcohol. Some of my dear friends are in recovery and I see their struggles and I'm amazed at the strength they have. What I'm about to say does not in any way diminish their fight. But in some ways being addicted to food is worse. Human beings can learn to live without drugs and alcohol, but we cannot learn to live without food. It's biologically impossible.

People who battle a food addiction must do so several times each day. Every time those of us who have battled this addiction eat. Every time food gets mentioned in a conversation. Or in the media. Every time a commercial comes on TV. Every time we pass a restaurant on the street. Food, quite simply, is everywhere, and therefore so is temptation. If you think this sounds overly dramatic, then congratulate yourself. Your relationship with food is probably healthier than mine ever was. I fought a war of wills each time I saw something edible on a plate. And always I fought this war alone, because—as I said—being fat carries a stigma. Most people like to generalize. They think that fat people are lazy or weak or passionless or worse. So even though you might be giving everything you've got to fight your addiction, you often do so without getting any support (or very little at any rate).

This uphill climb, this day-to-day stress, is hard on the person who wants to lose weight. But it also takes an incredible toll on their families and their friends. I know, because I lived through it, and so did the people close to me.

When I was growing up, my parents felt very conflicted about keeping treats in the house. It's normal for a kid to enjoy something sweet now and then, isn't it? A cookie or some cake, for example. Maybe a bowl of ice cream. But my parents were torn (of course they were—remember the Scale Fix Incident?). They wanted me to eat healthier foods because I was their son and they loved me and clearly I was fat. On the other hand, they didn't want to deprive me of anything. What would a childhood be like without some treats in moderation? What should they do?

The whole thing came to a head over something I now call Twinkie-Gate. Twinkies were one of my favorite treats. My mother used to buy them at the grocery store, along with those little chocolate cupcakes that come in pairs wrapped in cellophane. You know the kind I'm talking about—the ones with the dollop of whipped cream inside. Man, did I love Hostess!

Well, one day while I was still pretty young, I came home from school and snuck into the kitchen. This wasn't an easy thing to do because I was really, really big back then. When I moved around, the house creaked.

My mom kept the Twinkies in a drawer by the sink, and this drawer made an awful squeaking noise each time you pulled it open, which meant that it was nearly impossible to sneak anything out. But somehow I managed, mostly because Twinkies were great motivation. I pulled the drawer open and snatched up the Twinkies and pushed the drawer closed, putting all my effort toward making sure that I made no sound whatsoever. Then I snuck back as fast as I could to my room. Fat Kid Takes Up New Career as Cat Burglar. Film at eleven!

To this day, I don't know what was running through my head. Seriously, how did I think I was going to get away with it? My mother and I were the only two people in the house that afternoon. Sooner or later, she was bound to notice the box of Twinkies was empty. As it turned out, she stopped me right before I got to my room. She looked down and noticed the two Twinkies that were sort of hanging out of my pants pocket. Mom made me put the Twinkies back in the drawer, and I did. But then I went to back to my room and waited until I thought the coast was clear and snuck back out to the kitchen again and worked the drawer open carefully, carefully . . .

Wouldn't you know it? She caught me again. And this time she got angry. This woman who loved me so much, this woman whom I miss every day, had a look of anger on her face. Anger mixed with sadness and hurt.

I was just a kid at the time, maybe ten or eleven. But I still remember that look on her face. The pain in her eyes is still hard to describe, though it's easier to recognize now that I've gotten older. My mother wasn't upset that I was lying to *her*. She was more upset that I was lying to *myself*.

Looking back, I can see it so clearly. My weight was as much of a burden to my family as it was to me. More so, when you got right down to it, because I was in denial. But now I recognize the situation I put them in, the anxiety they had to endure, the decisions I forced them to make. They were so concerned about me. They also felt so powerless. Mom and Dad certainly weren't experts on fitness and nutrition, but they knew that a fat kid who tried to steal Twinkies every day was headed for all sorts of problems. And the agony I put them through didn't end there. They had to endure a whole lot more as they watched me go through life always being ostracized by my peers. My mother was the person who day after day saw me all alone. My parents understood something that I did not: that I was a prisoner, locked in my body, not comfortable with myself. They loved me with everything they had, but they couldn't set me free.

I know you probably know this already, and I don't mean to harp. But I seriously want you to consider this if you haven't done so before. *Our weight is an addiction, and like any addiction, it robs us of life and fulfillment of our potential.* Like any addiction, it always leads to massive personal suffering. And that suffering isn't ours alone. It spreads out, infecting our family and friends, those who are nearest and dearest to us, the people who love us the most. And if that's not a good enough reason to change, then I don't know what is.

Why Did I Write This Book?

When I first tried to lose weight, I looked all over the place for a guide, a set of instructions, some manifesto, *anything* that would inspire me and offer me common sense. I wanted a plan that I could follow, or maybe a friend who understood exactly what I was going through. A mentor. A coach. A teacher. A guide. And not just some pumped up exercise maven, but someone who *knew* what it was to be fat. Someone I could relate to.

Eventually I found the right group of people who helped to put my feet on the path to living fit and healthy. I'll tell you how that happened a little bit later on. But as far as a guide or instructions went . . . well, I looked everywhere, but it simply didn't exist.

Then, just a few years ago, I remembered that a wise man once said: *When you can't find the story you want to read, sit down and write it yourself.* And that's why I wrote this book. That's the purpose of *Fat Kid Got Fit*. Because, like I said, I think I know what you're feeling right now. You're frustrated. You want to change but you feel like the deck is stacked against you. And, like I was many years ago, you're probably operating under some colossal misconceptions.

For instance, you probably think that losing weight takes some Herculean act of will or some magnificent sum of money or something else you don't currently have. You probably think that you'll have to put in long hours at the gym. Hire a personal trainer or a talented surgeon. Buy some special machine advertised on TV (for five low payments of $39.95, shipping and handling not included). Maybe you think that it takes some special meal plan endorsed by popular TV stars. A magic potion. A special bracelet. Tapes that make you chant.

It doesn't. That's all incorrect. Regardless of how much weight you carry and how much you want to lose, you can start right now. In fact, you've *already* started. Wanting something is very important. It's the energy source that we'll tap like a well as we work to make your dream happen.

So why did I write this book? It's simple. *This is the book I wish I'd had when I was fat and just starting out on my journey.* This is the book that I needed to read, and so I wrote it.

Back on the Campaign Trail

Here's another fiasco I suffered. It's not quite as bad as TwinkieGate, but it's one that I'll always remember. One day, Chuck and I were visiting a senior citizens' center in Monmouth County, central Jersey, near the shore. Chuck gave his speech and the audience listened. When it ended, they applauded. Afterward, when the meeting broke up, I took a position standing by the refreshments table. That was always the best place to meet people, to talk with them and shake their hands. It also never hurt to be so close to the coffee and cookies.

An elderly woman walked up to me, smiling. I said hello and she reached right up and grabbed both my cheeks in both of her hands and pulled them apart like hunks of taffy. This woman pulled at my cheeks like she was trying to yank them right off my face.

"You have such a handsome face," she said. "You know that? If you'd just lose weight."

I was shocked. No, I take that back. I was utterly mortified. What this woman had said was a backhanded compliment under any circumstances, but I didn't even *know* her. *How dare she?* I thought. *How dare she say such a thing to me in a public place? In front of all these people?!?*

My defenses had taken over, of course. They were thinking for me and talking for me. Instead of hearing the "handsome" part, I just heard "lose weight." And yes, there was a certain irony involved. Like I said, I wanted a career in politics. In other words, I hoped to spend my life in front of the public, serving the public. But here I was getting angry that someone had used the public as a forum to state something so obvious. This woman was more outspoken than most, but she wasn't pointing out anything that people weren't probably thinking already. I couldn't hide.

This woman had skipped the gristle and meat and cut right down to the bone. I stood there, not knowing what to say. She smiled at me and patted my cheek, then turned and walked away. Looking back, I think I understand what she was doing. She was leaving me with a challenge. She was asking me who I wanted to be: a person who was healthy and fit, or a person who was not.

I hemmed and hawed and tried to shrug off what happened. I told myself that the woman was rude. She must have been out of her mind, I thought. Then I made myself get back to work. It was yet another wakeup call, but back then, I wasn't listening. My weight had dulled my sense of myself.

About two weeks after my heart attack scare in the men's room at the Pegasus restaurant, Chuck and I were back at the Meadowlands, only this time at the Sheraton Hotel. Chuck had a meeting scheduled with Bob DeCotiis. Bob was the chief counsel for Jim Florio, who had been governor of New Jersey.

I knew the routine, of course. While Chuck and Bob were having their talk, I set up shop at the hotel bar, doing paperwork, checking messages. But the situation filled me with an eerie kind of dread. Here I was back at the Meadowlands, and here I was leaving Chuck to do his thing while I stepped aside and went to the bar, exactly the same way I had before when the chest pains suddenly struck. I'd been certain I was dying then, but here I was in a similar spot, moving through nearly the same routine. I'd been given my second chance at life, but already two long weeks had passed and I hadn't done a single thing about it.

But then a very strange thought occurred to me. I thought:

I'm not doing anything about my condition because I don't know what to do*!*

Sure, I needed to lose some weight, but no one had ever taught me how. Clearly, the stuff I'd learned in high school health class wasn't cutting the mustard or mayo. Nor were the exercises I'd learned in phys ed. All the jumping jacks, squat thrusts, mountain climbers, and dodgeball games in the world weren't going to put a dent in my weight (as if I still played such games).

And things hadn't gotten much better in college. If anything, they had gotten worse. In college, I'd focused on studying hard, going out with my friends, and parties and drinking and that sort of thing. In other words, I'd focused on ignoring my weight as best I could. But where did that leave me? Fat, that's where. Fat and getting fatter.

Maybe there's some magic pill, I thought. *Some diet I haven't tried.*

I'd watched TV, like everyone else. I'd seen those infomercial gurus who spent their thirty-minute spots shouting about some magic machine they'd created to help people peel off the pounds. Some super-secret commando pushup you could learn from a videotape or a series of DVDs. Yes, there were solutions out there, but which one really *worked*? I didn't know, and not knowing made me feel helpless. Feeling helpless on top of fat is a very bad combination.

I stood at the bar, wrapped in my thoughts until I noticed that Chuck was just about finished. The meeting was over. He got up from the table and shook hands with Bob DeCotiis. That was my cue, so I went over and shook hands with Bob, as well. Then Chuck and I left the hotel.

We walked out into the parking lot and angled toward the Chuck Wagon. I remember it was a bright blue afternoon in early fall and neither of us said a word. Election Day was coming up fast. The polls said the race was neck and neck. I'm pretty sure Chuck and I were both wondering the same thing. *What happens next? Where do we go from here? Will all the hard work we've put in pay off? Has our sacrifice been worth it?*

We had a few more stops to make that day, and I was running through the itinerary in my mind when Chuck said, apropos of nothing, the words that would change my life.

"Wow. He looks great."

I snapped back to myself. "Huh?" I said. "Who's that?"

"Bob. It's unbelievable. Can't believe it's the same guy."

"What do you mean?" I said. "What happened?"

The tone of Chuck's voice was so reverential, so awestruck, I wondered if Bob had just suffered a heart attack. Or maybe he'd just learned to walk again after a terrible, debilitating accident. You'd probably have wondered these things yourself. Bob certainly *looked* normal enough to me—a pleasant, silver-haired guy in his fifties, tall and pretty trim . . .

"He lost a lot of weight," said Chuck. "I mean, he lost a *lot* of weight."

It was one of those *aha* moments in life, the kind where you wonder, *Is someone up there, reading my mind? And if so, are they trying to tell me something?*

We reached the Chuck Wagon, pulled the doors open, and got inside. I buckled myself into the driver's seat and tried to sound as nonchalant as possible when I asked, "Lost a lot of weight, huh? Really? How did he do it?"

Chuck had already grabbed the clipboard that held our itinerary sheet. He was scanning it to see where we were headed next. "Hmmm?" he mumbled, distracted. "How what?"

It embarrassed me to repeat what I'd said, but I did it. "How did he lose the weight?"

Chuck nodded, still reading. "Oh. He—ah—said something about going to Duke University."

"Really," I said, then nodded like that made perfect sense. But it didn't, of course. Not really. Bob DeCotiis was a lawyer, I knew. Why would he go back to school to learn how to lose weight? Was such a thing even possible?

I honestly didn't think so. Like I said, I'd gone to George Washington University, and I didn't recall hearing anything about courses in losing weight. Did people major in something like that? Could you maybe declare it a minor? I was suddenly, deeply, incredibly curious.

"Huh," I said. That was all that I said, but I made an important mental note. One that now, after all these years, I'm certain saved my life.

I keyed the ignition and hit the gas. The Chuck Wagon gave a tired groan and shuddered and started to roll. I aimed it toward the highway again and swung us into traffic. Chuck and I had places to be. We had to stay on schedule.

A Very Important Phone Call

'd only met Bob one time, but I got his number from Chuck Haytaian, called him up the very next day, and reintroduced myself. He said of course he remembered me and asked what was on my mind. This became the tricky part, the part where I had to commit.

I told Bob I hoped I wasn't asking him an offensive question, but I'd heard that he'd recently lost some weight and wondered how he had done it.

Bob laughed. "Offended?" he said. "Bill, I'm not offended at all."

I suddenly felt relieved. "Chuck mentioned you'd gone somewhere," I said. This next part sounded silly to me, but I asked it anyway. "You . . . ah . . . studied at some university?"

Bob laughed again. "Well, yes and no. I went to the Diet & Fitness Center at Duke University."

I'd heard of that famous school, of course, but I'd never heard of anything called the Diet & Fitness Center. Bob gave me their number and urged me to call, and I have to confess, I got really excited. Because even though I knew very little, I'd already started to get the impression that there was a place where people like me could go, a place where someone could teach me how to lose weight. A school for people who wanted to change.

Part of my excitement at that point was due to the fact that I'd always been good at school. I liked to study and learn new things. And Bob seemed so certain when he talked to me, so confident. Plus, whatever he'd done had clearly worked. I remembered how impressed Chuck was by the weight that Bob had lost. So I made the decision right then and there: *If Bob can do it, so can I.* What more did I really need than that?

Feeling excited, I thanked Bob for his time and hung up the phone. Then I picked it back up and called the number for Duke.

A woman answered and said hello and introduced herself as Barbara Dean. Have you ever met someone who's the very soul of Southern politeness? The kind of person who's so genuinely kind and hospitable they can put you at ease right away? That's Barbara Dean in a nutshell.

I introduced myself to Barbara and told her I'd just been talking about the Diet & Fitness Center with someone who'd attended. I told Barbara I was very interested in what went on at the center and wanted to know more about it. For instance: How could I get there? Where would I stay? Where would I eat? What would a typical day be like? How many people attended at once and how did they range in age—that sort of thing.

Barbara and I talked for about twenty minutes. She was very patient with me. I remember being most impressed by the fact that she didn't speak hype. She wasn't trying to sell me on anything—she really listened to me and really answered my questions. I appreciated that.

I told Barbara how much I weighed, and she recommended a four-week stay at the clinic. "It's the best thing for first time participants," she said. "A four-week stay will really allow you the time and opportunity to begin forming new strategies and lifestyle habits."

I remember thinking, *Lifestyle, huh?* What could a lifestyle possibly have to do with losing weight? Even though it didn't make sense to me at that moment, I gathered the word was important, so I took a mental note.

Barbara and I started talking about how much the Duke program would cost. I thought that a four-week package would end up being pretty expensive considering everything Barbara said was included. And it *was* expensive, about $4,000 at the time. Remember, I was a political aide, a job not renowned for its salary. Four thousand dollars would have been tough for me to swing under any normal circumstances. But I'd saved a lot of money while driving for Chuck Haytaian. One of the good things about eating so many political dinners is that you spend a lot less on food (my late night binges notwithstanding). I had some cash that was sitting in a savings account while I searched for a way to invest it. Law school had seemed like the most likely place.

But this is important, too, I thought. Maybe much *more* important.

I want to pause here and point something out, something I think you should really consider. *From early on, I saw going to Duke as an investment I would make in myself.* Call it a purchase of shares in stock of the life I'd always wanted. Besides, I thought, if I don't lose weight—and fast—I might not be around when it's time to collect any dividends.

Now let me be clear: I'm not saying you have to go to Duke to make this kind of investment. But I do recommend that you view your own path in very similar terms. *Everything you do to get fit is part of your personal journey. Own it. Demand the best from it. Demand the best from yourself.*

I remembered that awful moment in the men's room at the Pegasus restaurant. How could I not? Thinking of that, and remembering how it felt to look at myself in the mirror . . . to believe with all my heart that I was dying without ever having really lived . . . it was just too much to take. I told myself I was never going back to that place again. Not ever. I wasn't talking about the Pegasus, of course. I was talking about how I'd been that day. The state of body and mind I was in. I was talking about being fat and low, unhealthy and depressed.

"So when do you think you would like to come down?"

I was still on the phone with Barbara Dean. I pushed myself to focus a bit and thought the matter over.

"I'll have to get back to you on that," I said. She said that she'd send me some information about the Diet & Fitness Center. I thanked her and hung up the phone.

Election Day was coming up fast. We still had four or five months to go, but four or five months rocket past when you're running a very close race. The polls kept showing us neck and neck with the incumbent. We would have to work hard and never let up. My job until Election Day would demand my total focus. But I made a deal with myself. *If Chuck wins the Senate race*, I thought, *I'll go with him to Washington. I'll set up his office and work as his aide and deal with my weight issues then.*

Was I fooling myself? Of course I was. Did I really think I'd have time to lose weight while working as a senator's aide in the heart of the nation's capital? It was another convenient, colossal delusion, but that didn't matter to me. I told myself that I had no choice. If Chuck won the race, I would *have* to go. I'd be foolish to turn down a job like that. I'd worked super hard to help Chuck win. I'd *earned* the right to be at his side, to start the career I had dreamed of for years. My health? Who cared about that?

But of course, I thought, there's another side to this coin. If Chuck doesn't win, then I've made my decision. I would put myself through the program at Duke. I would finally confront my weight and see which one of us owned my life.

A Random Fat Kid Memory

Heavy or not, and car accidents aside (even despite my lingering fears of the dreaded pool and the pommel horse), I really started to change in high school. My work in the congressman's office had certainly helped to open me up. Plus, I got involved in the school musical, where I met lots of people I liked. Then I ran for president of my junior class and won, which made me feel great. Suddenly, I was popular. I was the guy in charge. And that meant that I had a ton of responsibilities, many of which began to overlap in interesting ways.

For instance, while rehearsing for the school show (that year it was *South Pacific*), I was also in charge of organizing the junior prom. So between rehearsals, I drove to the local German American Club, the space we had booked for the big event. I knew the people who worked at the club and they knew me from political functions I'd attended there over the years. I'd work my tail off on table arrangements and decorations, making sure that the favors came in on time. Making sure that the DJ was booked and knew where to set his equipment up. Making sure that the bills were paid, that everything ran smoothly. I'd glance at my watch and wouldn't you know it? Incredibly, my time would be up. I was due back at rehearsals again, so I'd drive back to school and park in the lot and run to the dressing room, get into costume, and hustle my big body out on the stage singing "There Is Nothin' Like a Dame!" at the top of my lungs. On top of all that, there were classes and clubs and the looming specter of SATs. And my work for the congressman's office, too. In all, it was a busy spring.

Somewhere in all this running around, it hit me that I hadn't asked anyone to be my date for the prom. So I asked a girl from my homeroom.

Her name was Jennifer. She was funny and she was also in the school show and she didn't have a date. So I asked her if she wanted to go. She said she'd think about it and get back to me. A few days later, she did, and her answer was no. That was strike number one.

I remember telling myself, *Don't take it so personally. This has nothing to do with you or your weight.* Yeah, right.

The second girl I asked was a friend of mine named Terry. We'd hung out a lot with friends that year, but Terry had recently twisted her ankle. She said that she didn't think she was going to go to the prom at all because of her injury. Fair enough. Remember, I was a fat kid. I'd heard stranger excuses before. Terry turned out to be strike number two.

Finally, I did one of the smartest things I've ever done in my life. I asked another girl whom I knew from the cast of *South Pacific*. Her name was Corinne Agins, and she was a sophomore at the time. Corinne said yes. Some enchanted evening, indeed!

So now I had my date for the prom. And now I felt really happy. But I'd waited so long to find a date that most of the table arrangements were full. So wouldn't you know it? Corinne and I ended up sitting with Jennifer, the first girl I'd asked, and her date, and Terry (whose ankle made a miraculous recovery) and the guy she ended up going with. Fat Kid Savors the Irony.

Really, it was no big deal. Everyone had a great time. But still, I remember how searing it felt. I'd be lying to say that it hadn't hurt, this ongoing sort of rejection. Here I'd finally made it out of my shell, finally reached a point in my life where I had a few friends I liked. My peer group knew who I was. I was president of my high school class and I liked that job; I liked doing things for people. It turned out I was good at it, too. But I was still a fat kid. Still getting rejected. Still being judged for my weight, not my worth. And that was tough. It really hurt to be judged by my body, by what I looked like, by the fact that I weighed as much as two or three of my peers put together.

One quick note about Corinne: She was (and still is) one of those very special people I hope it's your good fortune to meet in life. The kind who can see past what people look like to see who they really are. I would do anything for her, because of who she is and what she stands for in this world.

Interestingly, a number of years later when I was serving in the state legislature, Corinne called my office and asked for my help with an issue. I had a talented staff that was able to find many ways to help nearly all my constituents who called us with problems they needed solved. But we moved heaven and earth for Corinne. I would do it again if I had to. She still stands high in the pantheon of important people in my life, and for good reason. Sometimes I think of a world full of people like Corinne, and it never fails. I can't help but smile. A world like that—that would be something to see.

By the way, after I was elected to the legislature, I would march in our local Memorial Day parade each year. The procession would wind through the center of town and move down Nottingham Way past the house where Corinne and her family lived. And every year she'd run out in the street—she'd interrupt the whole darn parade—and call my name and throw her arms around me and give me a great big hug. People applauded and everyone cheered. The band would play, and nobody knew the link, I guess (or at least they didn't till now).

Corinne gave me hope when others did not. Encouragement when I needed it most. I doubt she understood how much that meant to me, then and now. Younger, older, fat, or fit, you never forget the people who choose kindness over cruelty.

Victory Pulled from the Jaws of Defeat

The Chuck Wagon burned out its engine in the final days of the long campaign. I suppose it had a decent excuse. In eleven months, Chuck Haytaian and I had put more than 110,000 miles on it. The heart of the Ford Econoline van just couldn't take anymore. One day it simply refused to start and that, as they say, was that.

Looking back, the van's demise presented a perfect metaphor. For one thing, it mimicked my own condition. Throughout the campaign I'd pushed myself hard, to the very brink and beyond. When things got tough, I told myself that I simply had to keep going, that silly distractions like how I felt and the state of my health and the weight of my body were nothing compared to winning the race and seeing Chuck get elected.

I remember I flip-flopped a lot back then. Yes, I'd made this deal with myself that I'd go to Duke if Chuck lost. But even after the heart attack scare, a part of me clung to the desperate illusion that I was overreacting somehow. That really my weight wasn't such a big deal. I was happy the way I was . . . wasn't I?

Basically, I'd gotten really good at lying to myself. I lied so well that I ended up believing the lies I was telling. Maybe you can relate to this.

But I call the Chuck Wagon's failed engine a perfect metaphor because it hinted at yet another sad defeat. On election night, November 8, 1994, after a long and arduous race, Chuck Haytaian lost to Frank Lautenberg, 47 percent to 51 percent.

It was one of those campaigns where everyone bit their nails to the quick right up to the very end. But the polls came in and the tallies were clear. Chuck had lost the election.

I remember feeling devastated, but Chuck seemed to take his defeat in stride. He went up to the front of our group and took the mic and gave his concession speech. He talked movingly about the direction he hoped New Jersey would take—under his watch, under anyone's watch. He thanked his staff for how hard we'd all worked. He thanked his supporters one and all.

I remember standing nearby as he spoke and feeling this incredible sense of disorientation. *Really?* I thought. *You mean . . . that's it? I don't have to wake up at five tomorrow morning and drive all over the state?*

In the campaign's closing weeks, my life had felt like a nonstop pendulum. On one side, there was my future in politics: a senator's aide in Washington. On the other side, there was North Carolina. A little far south of the Beltway, perhaps, and hardly the kind of work I'd envisioned, but that was totally inconsequential. A promise, after all, was a promise. It was time to go to Durham.

The next morning, after a buffet breakfast, I picked up the phone and called Barbara Dean and enrolled myself at Duke.

The Mystery of the Disappearing Me

These days, no one believes me when I tell this part of the story: I only told one person where I was going. Honestly. I didn't tell my colleagues. I didn't tell Chuck. I didn't tell even my closest friends. I told my father. Because I didn't want him to worry when his only son disappeared for a month.

My mother had recently passed away and I knew that my dad had a lot on his plate. But he listened very closely when I told him what I was planning to do. He didn't say a word throughout the whole explanation I gave.

I told him that my weight had always bothered me. This was a big admission, the first time I'd ever spoken those words to anyone on earth. I told him that I felt like my weight was holding me back from the best parts of life. I basically told him that I was unhappy. That's a hell of a thing for a father to hear from the mouth of his only son.

Dad didn't get upset or judge what I'd said or try to discuss it. He did what he's always done. He listened. It's one of the many reasons I love my dad so much. And when I finished, he nodded and shrugged and scratched his head and said, "How can I help?"

That's how my father has always been—100 percent supportive. He coached my Little League baseball team back when I could barely fit into my uniform. He always fought hard to get me involved with sports, with groups, with life. He's been on my side when no one else has been.

"I'll do whatever you need me to do," he said. "Just tell me what it is."

I thanked him, but told him that this was something I had to do on my own. Dad didn't get emotional. He didn't raise a stink. There wasn't any fanfare. He dealt with all of this matter-of-factly. I remember feeling so proud of that, that he trusted me to follow my instincts, to take a risk and try something new. His faith was like a shot in the arm, tripling my resolve.

Of course he asked some basic questions, like when did I plan to leave town? How long would I be gone? Just in case, he asked me to give him the address and phone number where I'd be staying. He asked me to call him now and again to tell him how things were going, and I promised him that I would.

But I didn't tell anyone else. Oh no. Absolutely not. I didn't want the pressure. After all, I could fail again. In choosing to send myself to Duke, I knew that I'd thrown down a very big gauntlet. The challenge I'd laid out for myself was bigger than any I'd ever attempted. I didn't want to disappoint anyone who might be rooting for me. If I went to Durham and lost some weight, I'd come back feeling victorious. But if nothing worked and I came back fat . . . then at least I had the option to continue to hide my shame.

I had no idea what the future would hold and, looking back, I was nervous. The way I saw it, my trip had two potential outcomes, and both seemed equally terrifying:

1. If I didn't lose weight, then I was a failure, fat for the rest of my life. I didn't want that to happen, of course, but failure almost seemed preferable to option Number Two, which was:

2. What if I really *did* shed the pounds? Who would I be then? I'd lived with my weight for twenty-two years. That's a very long time to get comfortable with a set of circumstances. Who was the person beneath all the fat? What kind of person would he be?

For the very first time in my life, I confronted a truth that I've now learned to take for granted. *Fear of failure is scary sometimes, but so is the fear of success.*

To get fit, I would effectively have to let my identity change. I'm sorry if that sounds somewhat dramatic, but trust me, it was the case. You probably know what I'm talking about. In fact, you probably already know the answer to my next and very important question, which is:

What Does It Mean to Be Fat?

Being fat can become a part of your identity, just like being an athlete can, or the fact that you play a musical instrument well, or the kind of job you do for a living, or being good at crossword puzzles.

When you're fat, you might be the jolly guy, the life of the party, everyone's friend.

When you're fat, you might be the smart kid who sits on committees but never gets up to dance at the prom. When it comes to sports, you're the team manager, or maybe the team statistician. Or umpire. You keep the score, but you're never a player, and certainly never a winner. Those roles all go to the people with grace, the jocks, the ones who jump high and fast and leave all the fat kids behind in the dust where we smile real big and pretend it's okay.

When you're fat, you're standing in front of the world. We're out in plain view—how can anyone miss us? They can't, of course. Because we're so big. But we're hiding a part of ourselves at the same time— or *parts* of ourselves, as the case may be. We laugh and we shrug. We apologize. We learn to restrict how we live our lives. To say things like, *Me? Oh no. I couldn't do that. It looks like fun, but I'm fat, you see? I'm sorry, it just wouldn't work . . .*

And by acting like this—with self-deprecation and modesty actually built upon shame—we keep from this world and everyone in it the gifts we could shower upon it instead. The world doesn't know what's inside of us, and probably never will. Because we have decided not to show it.

I want you to think about that for a moment. Really. Stop reading this book and think. I don't want to make sermons and it isn't my job to preach. But that, more than ever, is why you are here. I think that's the primary reason you first picked up this book. You have more to offer. You know that you do. And the world is waiting to take what you give. It's waiting with bated breath to receive the gifts you would like to bestow.

I hadn't figured any of this out when I first decided to lose my weight, to see what was underneath. But I know it now. And I want you to know: Getting fit is worth the trip. It helps you lead the kind of life you've always wanted to live.

I can't say what that means to you—it's a very personal question. Maybe it's being a better role model to your kids. Maybe it's being able to go for a long walk on a beach with someone special. Maybe it's the high you get when you set a physical goal for yourself, like running a mile or playing a game of basketball with friends. Maybe it's knowing your health is your wealth, and you won't have to worry so much anymore that your body could someday betray you. Any way you slice it, life is better when you get fit.

But I wasn't there yet. Not by a long shot. Old habits (especially the bad ones) can be awfully hard to break. As proof, I offer another story.

My Last Meal before Going to Duke

The day before I checked into Duke, I left New Jersey and drove south for four hundred miles. It was the Saturday after Thanksgiving and I'd eaten really well. I spent that night at a friend's place in Williamsburg, Virginia. Then, the next morning, Sunday, I got up very early and drove the remaining two hundred miles to Durham, North Carolina.

The opening session at the Diet & Fitness Center was scheduled to start at 6 p.m. Sunday night. I had booked myself into the apartments directly across the street from Duke. The place was very convenient and, since this was my first trip, the DFC staff had strongly suggested I stay there. Picture one of those hotel/apartment-type complexes for traveling businesspeople. You get a tiny one-bedroom apartment with a little living room and an efficiency kitchen. The entire place surrounds a pool—you know the kind of place I'm talking about.

I wanted to get there in plenty of time to check in and get my key and drop off my bags and make myself at home. Throw the suitcase onto the bed. Unzip the top and hang up some clothes. Go to the bathroom. Set up my toothbrush. Make sure the towels were clean. It seemed very important to get this just right because I already carried a sense that these next four weeks would be pivotal in my life. But before I got too far from Williamsburg, I pulled my car off the highway and hit a drive-through McDonald's.

I was on Route 85 and had just crossed the border into North Carolina. I wanted to eat a big, hearty breakfast because I faced a long day ahead and I told myself that I needed my strength. So I ordered two sausage biscuits with egg, two orders of hash browns, and one of those sugary orange drinks, which I super-sized, of course. Because, hey, I was a big guy, right? And big guys get really thirsty.

Now, I promise I'll never get technical with you when talking about food. Like I said, I'm not a nutritionist. I don't have a medical degree. You don't have to understand the role of hydrogen atoms in polyunsaturated fats in order to get fit. But I want you to look at the following stats and perform some simple addition. My hope is that you'll start to see how addition (and subtraction, too) are really the only tools you'll need to start losing weight, and fast.

Nutritional Information for 1 Sausage Biscuit with Egg

Calories	450
Calories from Fat	252
Total Fat	43% of daily intake based on a diet of 2,000 calories per day (daily value)
Cholesterol	260 mg or 87% of daily value
Sodium	930 mg or 39% of daily value

But remember, I ate *two* sausage biscuits the morning before I checked into Duke. Which means that my total intake that morning from Sausage Biscuits with Egg alone was:

Calories	900
Calories from Fat	504
Total Fat	86% of daily value
Cholesterol	520 mg or 174% of daily value.
Sodium	1860 mg or 78% of daily value

But hang on a minute. We're just getting started. Let's not forget the hash browns I ate. Here are the hash brown stats:

Nutritional Information for 1 Order of Hash Browns

Calories	147
Calories from Fat	83
Total Fat	14% of daily value

| Cholesterol | 0 mg or 0% of daily value |
| Sodium | 307 mg or 13% of daily value |

And of course, we have to double those values since I ate two orders of hash browns, as well . . .

Calories	294
Calories from Fat	166
Total Fat	28% of daily value
Cholesterol	0 mg or 0% of daily value
Sodium	614 mg or 26% of daily value

Lest we forget, there's still the little matter of my super-sized orange drink. My 42-ounce serving size amounted to this:

Calories	460
Calories from Fat	0
Total Fat	0% of daily value
Cholesterol	0 mg or 0% of daily value
Sodium	75 mg or 3% of daily value

So what does the food that I ate add up to?

Calories	1,654
Calories from Fat	670
Total Fat	114% of daily value
Cholesterol	520 mg or 174% of daily value.
Sodium	2549 mg or 107% of daily value

Now *that's* a great way to start your day! (I'm joking, of course.)

Like I said, you don't have to know anything about fats and saturated fats and trans fats and all that to get the point I'm trying to make. You just have to use your common sense. In fact, here's the simplest way to look at this breakdown: Check the final values. *Everything's over 100 percent!* My cholesterol intake practically *doubles* the daily value (which isn't a very good thing). So think of it like this:

If my body was a credit card, by eating this sort of meal in the morning, I'd already maxed it out. Actually, I'd maxed it out, applied for more credit, got it, and nearly maxed *that* out, too. And I still had the rest of the day ahead. Lunch and dinner and maybe a snack. Maybe a late night nosh . . .

You might be asking, *What were you thinking?* You might say, *But Bill! Didn't you* know *what you were* doing?

The honest answer? No, I didn't. Not really. Food to me was, well . . . food. I ate it when I got hungry and I never pondered it more than that. I thought that's what food was for. I also liked food you could get pretty quick because I was really busy (that's what I told myself, anyway)—I had to stay on the go. And yes, I loved how this fast food tasted. That was all the more reason to eat it, right? I mean, how could something that tasted so good be bad for you? That didn't make sense.

And as for the quantity? Well, like I said. I told myself I had a big day ahead. I had no idea what the Diet & Fitness Center would be like, so I needed to eat to keep up my strength and deal with whatever they asked of me. Also, there was the fact that eating a lot made me feel full, and feeling full made me feel happy. And happiness is important, right? Why be alive if you're not happy?

These are the games I played with myself, the illusions I chose to invest in. But before we go any further, are you starting to get the idea? By that, I mean specifically: Are you noticing any similarities between my old behaviors and yours?

Don't worry if you can't see them right now—it might take a while for things to sink in. I know it did with me. If it helps, I want you to know one thing: That breakfast I had at that roadside McDonald's? The one I just told you about? *That was the last time I ever ate fast food. Ever.*

When I finished eating breakfast, I pulled my car back onto the highway and kept heading south, toward Duke. There was no way I could have known it right then, but my life was about to begin.

The Big Moment Arrives

Hereafter, I'll refer to my first day at the Duke Diet & Fitness Center as The Day That Saved My Life. Because that's what it was, no question about it. That, and a whole lot more.

When I first arrived at Duke, I was twenty-two years old. To this day, I remain convinced that if I hadn't gone—right then, right there—I'd have never made it to thirty.

I don't remember the name of the woman who welcomed my little class. I do remember there were about ten of us from all over the country. Delores, who was from Texas, for instance. Chris, who was from New Jersey, like me. Nicole, who hailed from Florida. Our group pretty much comprised a cross-section of the country, as well as every age demographic. I think we bonded quite well, and fast, probably for the same reason so many people make lifelong friends during their freshman year at college. You start off as new faces in a new environment. Gradually, you put yourself out there, get to know each other. Realize you're all in the same boat together. And often you end up finding that you really like each other.

For that very first meeting, my group gathered in a conference room and introduced ourselves to one another and took seats around the big table. The atmosphere was relaxed and friendly, much more informal than what I'd imagined. The woman began to tell us what the next four weeks would be like. I don't remember everything she said verbatim, but I can paraphrase what got through to me during that orientation. One part sticks out sharply in my mind because it left me so flabbergasted.

What we teach you here is not a diet. Diets do not work.

When the orientation leader at Duke said this, it hit me like a brick in the face. I remember thinking, *Wait a minute . . . what do you mean diets don't work? How can that be?* Everyone who wants to lose weight tries a diet, right? And wasn't I at the Duke Diet & Fitness Center? Isn't that what they called the place? I turned my orientation binder over and read the name embossed on the front. Yup. It said so right there in big red letters: The Duke Diet & Fitness Center. Now I was very confused. But the staffer continued, and this is what I took from her words:

> *People who indulge in diet thinking will not lose weight—or not for long, at any rate. They may experience short-term victories, but their long-term prospects are horrible. They end up putting the weight back on. In fact, very often, they pack on more weight than they ever lost in the first place.*

This came as an absolute shock to me. It seemed as though I'd been operating under a major misconception. Up until that point, I'd figured that I could simply go to Duke, lose some weight, leave Duke, and go back to the life I had led before. Same life, only smaller. Thinner.

Wrong.

But the woman who was speaking continued, and this time she cleared up the problem:

> *Instead of teaching you how to diet, we will teach you to change your lifestyle.*

Aha! I thought. That word again! "Lifestyle" . . . Barbara Dean had said it. Now the orientation leader was saying it, too. Clearly this was important. I still didn't understand quite what she meant, so I listened very carefully. And the speaker continued:

> *This is not a spa. This is a workshop. Here you will learn to make something called a healthy lifestyle. We will provide you with tools and the knowledge required to use them. Our goal is not to do the work for you. Our goal is*

to prepare you so that you are the craftsman. You are the master. You are in charge. When you leave this place, you do so under your own steam, prepared to function on your own.

This wasn't what I'd expected, but still . . . it certainly didn't sound bad. Then the speaker dropped this bombshell. She told us (again, I'm paraphrasing):

Your weight is not an issue you will tackle for the next four weeks, or the next six months, or even the next six years. It's an issue that you will deal with throughout the rest of your life. And the rest of your life starts now.

"And remember," she said. "Ultimately our goal—and yours—is not to help you lose weight. Ultimately our goal is to help you live life to its greatest potential."

Aha! I thought. That's just what I want. My greatest potential, indeed!

Diet Thinking vs. Lifestyle Thinking

As our orientation leader kept talking, this notion of diet thinking versus lifestyle thinking began to clarify itself in my mind. I started to see how diet thinking is really a twisted form of logic, one that is doomed to fail from the start because of what it represents.

For instance, when you're in dieting mode, your thoughts might start to sound something like this:

> *I will starve myself! Yes! That's what I'll do! At the same time, I will work out like a mouse on a wheel! Yes! And then—even though I've exhausted myself and my body is crying out for food—I will starve myself again! Ha ha! I can already feel myself losing the weight!*
>
> *Because I'm on a diet, I won't listen to my body (ha ha!). Why would I do something silly like that? I know I've tried to diet before but this time I'm going to lose the weight! This time I'll keep it off for sure!*
>
> *This time I'll keep working out and restricting my food and working out until finally I drop the pounds!*
>
> *This time I'll make it work, do you hear?!? This time I'll absolutely 100 percent make it work and—oh, wait. Is that a cupcake?*
>
> *GIVE ME THAT CUPCAKE!*

The truth is, when we use diet thinking, we're really just lying to ourselves. It's exactly like that speaker told us my very first day at the DFC. Sure, we might win some short-term battles, but we lose the war in the long run. It's practically guaranteed.

Drastic measures often result in drastic changes for drastically short periods of time. And then, of course, there's the inevitable: the drastic backlash, the part where most dieters put back on all the weight they took off. Then take it off again. Then put it back on. And off and on and off and on like a yo-yo, out of control . . .

> *Hurray for me, I'm down fifteen pounds!*
> *Whoops. What's this? I'm up twenty-five.*
> *Wait. No no! Hold on for a second! I'm actually down seventeen!*
> *Oh darn. Look at this—I'm up twenty this month . . .*

Your body isn't the only thing getting pulled in all directions. Think of what this kind of living does to your self-esteem. It's up one day, shot down the next, attached to a number that shows on a scale. You exhaust yourself emotionally by running on a mental treadmill. Two steps forward, three steps back—day in and day out, month after month. A roller coaster of feelings.

With diet thinking, your emotions move in rapid succession. The triumph. The guilt. The pride. The self-loathing. The exultation. The angst. No wonder nobody likes to diet. Doesn't it sound like fun?

But look at the following list I've drawn up. Note how the very same goal—to get fit—can be handled very differently. All you have to do is make a very important shift . . . from Diet Thinking to Lifestyle Thinking. Please take note of the differences.

Who's in Charge?

With Diet Thinking, the diet's in charge. You must adhere. You have no choice. You stay on the diet or else you fall off. It's one or the other, a black and white issue. The diet is master. And this includes a fitness regime whose goals are usually out of reach. *Today, I'll start running five miles a day despite the fact that I've never run before!*

With Lifestyle Thinking, *you* are in charge. You decide what you want to eat according to what *you* like and what *you* know to be healthiest for you. You also decide when you want to eat according to the unique demands that are made by your highly specific schedule. With Lifestyle Thinking, there is no master. You and your body find ways to interact harmoniously, and this goes beyond the obvious spheres of diet and exercise. It permeates everything that you do, all aspects of your existence. And this harmonious interaction is never limited by a calendar.

Thinking Patterns

Diet Thinking is stubborn, uncompromising, and rigid. Everything you eat has to be a certain way, at a certain time, from a certain brand, with a certain count of fats, calories, proteins, and carbohydrates. Diet Thinking is disciplinary. Punishment figures prominently when you do or eat something that "isn't on the plan." A certain amount of self-loathing often accompanies Diet Thinking. Failure beckons, so diets end. Your thinking pattern tells you that you knew it would happen anyway. After all, you're just not good enough, right?

On the other hand, Lifestyle Thinking patterns are very loose and relaxed. It's okay if you substitute foods here and there, so long as it all adds up in the end to a pattern that maximizes your health. Yes, there are rules, but they're not so rigid—more like principles than rules. Principles are flexible while rules of course are not. With Lifestyle Thinking options always abound. Lifestyle Thinking can best be described as gentle, soft, and adaptable. Lifestyle Thinking is instructive without resorting to rancor. Well-planned, healthy rewards figure prominently when you've enjoyed a good stretch of doing or eating things that you know are healthy for you. (Though oftentimes, you'll decline this perk since health is its own kind of special reward.) A certain amount of self-respect goes hand in hand with Lifestyle Thinking. There really is no such thing as failure, so Lifestyle never ends. Diets are temporary. A lifestyle is forever.

Language Patterns

It's interesting that, as a person thinks, so does he or she speak. If you listen very carefully to how another person talks, you begin to see how their thoughts are constructed—and of course you can do this for yourself, as well.

A person engaging in Diet Thinking will often make highly critical, negatively grounded statements. For instance, if they eat a big meal, they might say, "I blew it, I'm off my diet again!" or "I'll never get this right!" Or they might beat themselves up, like this: "I should *never* have had that piece of cake! What on earth was I *thinking*?"

But a person who uses Lifestyle Thinking will choose a different vocabulary. Lifestyle statements still deal with the issues, but look ahead instead of backwards, and always with a supportive tone, always with a gentle conviction. For instance a Lifestyle Thinker might say, "Okay, well, I splurged tonight. We're back on track tomorrow." Or they might ask themselves questions that delve toward the root of the experience. "I wonder why I ate more than I'd planned to tonight. What could have triggered that? How can I plan around that trigger in the future?"

Another interesting point about language patterns is that they can take place both externally and internally. External talk is what we say, but internal talk is what we think. Both are powerful. Lifestyle Thinkers learn to monitor both. When necessary, they adjust their vocabulary to help them get more out of life.

Progress and Self-Worth

With Diet Thinking, you measure your progress by how many pounds you've lost, and *only by how many pounds you've lost*. Therefore, until you meet your goal weight (that precious number you've got in your head), your self-worth amounts to very little, and sometimes even worse. With Diet Thinking, you see yourself as nothing until you get thin. There's also this very misguided notion that once you get thin, you stop. You've won! (Nothing could be further from the truth.)

With Lifestyle Thinking, you measure your progress by how good you feel about yourself. You focus on activities and foods that give you energy and inspire you to be the best version of yourself you can possibly be. Weight loss is actually secondary, a by-product of good practice. You honor yourself at the very beginning and throughout the entire process, not just as a reward for when you finally attain some arbitrary goal. With Lifestyle Thinking, every tiny step you make along the journey is a cause for celebration. And fitness under a Lifestyle Plan is an ongoing thing, a long relaxing walk on a beach instead of a sprint down a tight dark tunnel.

Attitudes toward Food

With Diet Thinking, food becomes evil, the source of all temptations. Diet Thinkers can't think about food without engendering confrontation. You develop a deep resentment toward some foods because you think, "I can't have those, they'll pull me off my diet and make me pack on the pounds again!" To keep yourself from backsliding, you struggle constantly to bolster your willpower to superhuman levels where (since no one is superhuman) you're setting yourself up to fail.

With Lifestyle Thinking, you understand and embrace the properties all foods possess. You select the foods you'll enjoy eating based on how they affect your overall health instead of on fulcrums of guilt or need or shame or misery. With Lifestyle Thinking, you never develop resentments toward food because *it's all about finding a balance.* So you make informed choices to put your body on the path to wellness. You even splurge every now and then by giving yourself a treat. With Lifestyle Thinking, food is your ally. You work together to live healthfully.

Attitudes toward Feeling Full

With Diet Thinking, hunger pangs get tied to deep-seated emotions and behavioral triggers. Stress can make you feel empty, which makes you hungry, which leads to blind, compulsive, self-destructive eating behaviors. The same can be said of exercise, or the disastrous lack thereof. Diet Thinking often says, "I'm too tired to go for a walk" or "I've had a bad day, so it's time to slack off." A Diet Thinker often cannot tell the difference between a physical need and a craving of the spirit.

Lifestyle Thinking treats hunger more as a symptom than a condition. When people who practice Lifestyle Thinking feel hungry, they assess what they've eaten lately to see if they're due for more food. If food is required, they eat just enough to keep their bodies running at maximum levels given their rates of activity: no more, no less. Lifestyle Thinkers always factor emotional conditions into their hunger pangs. If they feel like they really *have* to eat something, they substitute with healthy alternatives that add to their feelings of wellness. And while many cases exist when a person is too exhausted to exercise, Lifestyle Thinkers know that the antidote to a challenging day or a trying situation often lies in a brisk walk or jog, an exercise class at their local gym, or a physical game they can play with friends to increase their sense of belonging.

Attitudes toward Exercise

Diet Thinking treats exercise as a terrible chore that must be performed. Diet Thinkers literally attack their exercise. They grunt, they groan, they scream, they're dramatic. They love to rattle off slogans like "no pain, no gain" or "gotta get pumped" or "time to kick some butt!" With Diet Thinking, you punish yourself for the sin of eating and enjoying it. Your body is something to be hewn, broken, crushed, blasted, castigated, blown apart. If you listen very closely, you'll hear a lot of Diet Thinkers express these attitudes in their daily vocabulary.

On the other hand, Lifestyle Thinking treats exercise as a catalyst toward your quality of life. In other words, the more fit you are, the more energy you'll have. With Lifestyle Thinking, you take exercise as a way of charging your batteries up instead of burning them out. With Lifestyle Thinking, exercise is regarded as fun, a privilege, a way to unwind. Going to the gym isn't a chore or a punishment. Lifestyle Thinkers also know to vary their forms of exercises to keep the experience fresh.

A final word on the difference between Diet Thinking versus Lifestyle Thinking. Aristotle once said, "We are what we repeatedly do. Excellence, then, is not an act, but a habit." Habit is the key word here. Think about your habits for a moment. Then ask yourself this:

- Given what I've just read, how am I prone to think? In Diet terms or in Lifestyle terms?

- Looking back with this new information, how am I prone to act? As a Diet Thinker or Lifestyle Thinker? (Try to be honest here.)

If either of the questions above led you to think you've been doing things wrong, fear not. That's what this journey is all about. A wiser person than me once said that knowing exactly what problem you face is 90 percent of discovering an appropriate solution.

Remember, we're here to explore the way you've been thinking, and how that thinking has led to your actions, which in turn have formed habits. Once we find healthier ways to think, we'll get to decide which actions best correspond with these new Lifestyle Thinking patterns. Then we'll practice and practice these actions until they become strong habits. Better habits than what we've been using. Habits that help us to get and stay fit.

So let me take a moment to recap. Diet Thinking and Lifestyle Thinking—that's the first thing I learned at Duke, and for me it clicked immediately. The lightbulb went on, the stars aligned, call it whatever you will. Basically, what I understood was this: *I'd been thinking wrong and acting wrong, and trying to lose my weight the wrong way.* In fact, I'd fallen headfirst into a trap that was set by my ignorance.

For example, I'd truly come to believe those outrageous claims made by the diet industry. And this, more than anything, had to be dealt with. But first, let's review what they want you to think.

What the Diet Industry
Doesn't Want You to Know

The diet industry is a business. They seek to sell things and make profits.

The product could be a piece of gym equipment. Or a "juicer" that's really a glorified blender with lots of fancy lights on the front that blink whenever you turn it on. It could be one of those padded coils you squeeze between your thighs. It could be a vitamin supplement or a workout video or a pack of cards that you deal out every day to reach a healthier you. It could be that slimming grapefruit regime used by your favorite Hollywood stars. Some sources estimate that Americans spent $58 billion on these products in 2010 and forecast that the industry will probably continue to grow by 6 percent a year until it reaches a cap of $68.7 billion per annum.[10]

Frankly, it doesn't matter what the product is. Why? Because none of them are designed to educate you in proper nutrition. None of them are designed to teach you simple, effective exercises that get your body fit and keep it that way for life. None of them deal with you as a person—your issues, your habits, and your beliefs. They're gimmicks, worthless baubles and trinkets specifically designed to appeal to those of us who are mired in Diet Thinking.

If I just eat this specialty diet food or use this amazing slimming machine, I'll finally once-and-for all get thin and then I can stop all this diet nonsense . . .

All that glitters isn't gold. How many of these companies and manufacturers maintain long-term studies on their Magic Machine or their special Acai berry–based bars or their martial arts–inspired exercise video? How many of them disclose the percentage of people who actually lose weight for good by using their technique or product? The answer is zero. The reason? Simple.

These companies and manufacturers know that there's nothing inherently wrong with the product they're selling. Some people buy it, try it, get fit. They feel pretty good for a couple of weeks, maybe even a couple of months. But most of them soon fall back to the patterns they had before making their purchase.

These companies know that most American consumers won't use their product or technique for life. Nor do they care, not one darn bit. They simply want your money. They're riding the wave of your impulse shopping, hoping to be the next product you buy (sent to you, shipping and handling included, but only for a limited time!). They're hoping to provide you with the latest, most amazing fitness gimmick . . . until the next paycheck comes along and flies right out of your bank account.

These companies and manufacturers know the real secret to getting fit, and it has nothing to do with their products at all. It has to do with *lifestyle*.

These companies know what I'm going to teach you: All you need is some common sense and a vision of who you want to be. And the rest— the part where you drop excess weight, build muscle, and start to enjoy your life (I call this getting fit, by the way—that's exactly what getting fit means) . . . well, that starts to happen all by itself. And because you like the lifestyle you planned, it sticks around. Not for a week and not for a month. Again: It's for the rest of your life.

You don't believe me? That's okay. I sympathize, I really do. I didn't believe it either when I first attended Duke. But there's a sinister sort of disparity between what the diet industry wants you to think and what their products actually do . . . and again, the fulcrum of this disparity rests on one thing: money. *Your* money in *their* pockets.

I'll give you the best example I know, one that I hope will set the right tone. Let's talk about diet soda.

The Diet Soda Myth

Some people go crazy for diet soda. They act like it's the fountain of youth or something, a silver bullet for losing weight, the perfect solution.

Everyone knows people who go out to dinner and order an appetizer of pasta Alfredo with a dozen fried shrimp and then a 48-ounce steak with fries, then cheesecake with two scoops of chocolate ice cream and peanut brittle on top for dessert. And they sit there wolfing this big meal down while drinking a diet cola. Because (they'll tell you guiltily), sure, they're shooting the moon that night (you can read this as "breaking their diet"). But they're actually really and truly committed to trying to lose some weight.

Okay, I admit it: *I* used to do that. I used to engage in this magical thinking that diet soda would help me lose the pounds no matter what else I was eating. In fact, I used to think that I could drink diet soda day in and day out because there aren't any calories in diet soda, right? And zero calories means I won't put any weight on. Right?

Uh-uh. Wrong.

Don't believe this zero calorie = no weight story. It's just that: a story. It's an advertising hook designed to make you feel good enough about a product so that you'll invest in it. Sadly, the truth is a lot more complicated.

Drinking soda (yes, even diet soda) can't help you lose weight. In fact, a lot of new studies show that even the zero-calorie drinks can be very bad for your health. How? *They might not supply any calories but they can still condition you to seek out poor food choices.* What does that mean? I'll tell you.

Diet sodas taste sweet, right? Of course they do. Nobody wants to drink something that tastes like a hot cup of salt. But to maintain a zero-calorie count, these diet sodas use artificial sweeteners, *many of which have been shown to prime or condition our palates to makes us seek sweet foods.*

What's a sweet food? Here's another place where people tend to get fooled. I'm not just talking about cupcakes and candy bars (though yes, those treats are included). I'm talking about breads and cereals, too. I'm talking about any food that's high in carbohydrates because carbohydrates are sugars.

So okay, maybe it's technically true: You're not consuming any calories when you drink a diet soda. But the appetite you develop soon after—the one that drives you to eat a massive bowl of pasta as a snack, or a whole box of chocolate chip cookies—*that* can really pack on the pounds, and a lot of new research points to the fact that appetites like this increase from drinking diet soda.

ABC News did an exposé in 2007 based on a study by the National Heart, Lung, and Blood Institute of the National Institutes of Health. The study stated that as little as one can of soda a day can correlate to a 48 percent increased risk for "metabolic syndrome," sometimes known as insulin resistance. Another researcher in the 1970s noted that metabolic syndrome leads to a "constellation of abnormalities" that go beyond heart disease and obesity and strike at the core of the aging process, as well as other clinical states.[11]

But one of the most shocking studies was presented on the opening day of the International Stroke Conference in Los Angeles in February 2011. Conducted by the University of Miami's Miller School of Medicine, the study followed 2,564 residents of Manhattan for nine years and gathered data on their eating and exercise habits, cigarette and alcohol use, blood pressure, cholesterol levels, and so on. At the end of the testing, researchers concluded that people who drank diet soda every day had a 61 percent higher risk level for "vascular events" (a term that includes heart attacks and strokes) over those people who drank no diet sodas at all.[12]

The researchers in this study admitted that their results could be caused by something they missed in their work, some factor that drinkers of diet soda possess that has nothing to do with diet soda. But frankly, I doubt that's the case. Earlier testing on animals suggests a link between vascular problems and the caramel coloring used in dark-colored sodas like colas.

And here's another reason why diet sodas can be bad for you: They contain high levels of sodium, which causes high blood pressure . . . which causes bloating, and can also cause heart disease while increasing your risk of diabetes, stroke, and other disorders such as gout and calculi ("stones" in the kidney and bladder and several other places besides). You can think of it sort of like this: You drink a soda to lose some weight and increase your dosage of salt . . . salt has been known to make people thirsty, which often inspires them to reach for . . . guess what? *Another diet soda!*

This vicious circle I'm talking about gets even worse when the beverage you drink contains a ton of caffeine. Because caffeine, of course, can be very addictive. And maybe it starts to explain why U.S. consumers spent $21 billion on "low-calorie" beverages in 2007. And by the way, abundant caffeine consumption has also been clinically proven to make people uptight, anxious, and sleep-deprived—so add that into the list.

One researcher for ABC, Dr. David L. Katz, was also associated with the Yale Medical School and the Yale Prevention Research Center. He's the health columnist for the *New York Times* Syndicate and the nutrition columnist for *O, The Oprah Magazine*. Dr. Katz took his comments on soda intake to an even more poignant level. He said that sodas contain strong doses of acid, which, when consumed in high quantities (twelve cans of soda a day, for instance), can start to impact the health of our bones, ruining them prematurely. Twelve cans of diet soda a day was something I often indulged in before I went to the Duke DFC. Sure, to me, that's ancient history. But now I wonder: What about you?

Do you still think I'm overreacting? I recently read an article by Katherine Zeratsky, a dietician with the Mayo Clinic. She says that one glass of soda a day probably can't hurt us (moderation, as we'll find out, is the key to enjoying most things in life). But more than one serving of soda a day, she says—be it regular or diet—increases our risk of obesity, heart problems, and type 2 diabetes.

Have you ever heard *that* in a soft drink commercial? Of course not, and I bet you know why. I can't speak for the soft drink companies of the world, but don't you think they'd be really upset if the general population started to equate obesity, heart problems, high blood pressure, kidney and bladder stones, melting skeletons, restless nights, substance addiction, and type 2 diabetes with the products they're trying to sell us?

In the very same *ABC News* exposé, a spokesman for Coca-Cola North America was asked to comment on the research being presented. Her response? "Great taste. No calories. Wholesome ingredients. How could you drink too much?"[13]

But then, as Ms. Zeratsky notes, why should we drink soda at all? Yes, an occasional treat is fine (the operative word is *occasional*, which goes back to moderation again). How about a hydrating glass of water with a squirt of lemon and cranberry juice? I guess the question I'm trying to ask is: Why not develop new habits that are both enjoyable and healthy?

I'm not saying that you should never drink diet soda. Saying never is part of Diet Thinking, remember? However, I am saying that healthier alternatives to diet soda exist. And I am saying it can't hurt to limit your diet soda intake to reach your overall fitness goals. This kind of common-sense-to-fitness approach is what led me to develop my Fit Tips.

Wait! What the Heck Is a Fit Tip?

I t's exactly what it sounds like: a simple bit of advice that's easy to com-prehend, easy to use, and easy to plug right into your lifestyle without any huge interruptions or drama. Unless you're the type who really needs drama. In which case, I can't help you.

Getting fit can be simple to do, provided you really want it. These tiny bits of good advice will help you to get fit and stay that way. I've sprinkled them throughout this book wherever their topics seemed most appropriate. You don't need to worry about remembering them. Most of them make such perfect sense, they're bound to stick in your mind. I've also listed them all in the back of this book. Tear out the page and make a few copies. Post one in your office space and one in your kitchen at home. Read it to yourself every day—that will help you a lot! Let that list and everything on it become a big part of your daily routine. Let it shape (dare I say the word?) your brand new fitness *lifestyle*.

But let me be clear on this right from the get-go:

Fit Tips are *not* part of some wacky diet or crazy exercise program.

Actually, far from it.

They're common-sense ways to develop a lifestyle that lets you lose weight and get in shape and stay that way for the rest of your life.

Fit Tips are the same bits of wisdom I started to heed when I first made the choice to change my own life. I still follow them today, and for a simple reason: They work.

And so—without further ado—I offer my very first Fit Tip, which is:

Fit Tip #1: Almost Never Drink Soda

Yes, I mean diet sodas, too. In fact, I pretty much include all processed beverages in this list. Sodas and diet sodas, yes, but it also means sports drinks, energy drinks, and the great majority of the beverages sold as fruit drinks. Because a lot of these drinks aren't really made with fruit. They're mostly made of sugar.

I'm not trying to be a zealot here. If you don't believe this will help you lose weight, then try this simple four-part experiment:

Part One Walk into your local grocery store. Go to the beverage section and take a look at all the selections they have: sodas, diet sodas, sports drinks, iced teas, and so on. All the things I've mentioned above. Even the ones that claim to be healthy for you.

Part Two Pick up any one of these containers and flip it over. Start to read the list of ingredients. See how far you can get before you read something you can't pronounce.

Part Three Ask yourself if you know what that substance you can't pronounce really is (since you can't pronounce it, I'm betting you don't).

Part Four Now ask yourself why you're putting something like that in your body.

Look, this is hardly earth-cracking news, but processed drinks aren't necessarily as good for you as they say they are. My biggest pet peeve with processed drinks is the corn syrup they contain. Corn syrup is in practically everything these days. Companies use it as an artificial sweetener, a cheap synthetic substitute for actual cane sugar.

Little-known fact: They used to manufacture corn syrup by boiling corn in hydrochloric acid, which in turn was manufactured by passing salt over a mercury screen. Some of these elements are still reportedly present in corn syrup manufacturing.[14] Sound appetizing?

Granted, this method isn't used anymore; they phased it out a few years back. But the fact remains that corn syrup is nothing but empty sugar. It has no nutritional qualities. Combined with the fact that it's in practically every beverage I've listed above (along with other wacky ingredients), is it any wonder why so many of our bodies have begun to gain weight at such a rapid pace?

So Fit Tip #1 is easy: Almost never drink soda. At very least cut back on it. This is a simple step to losing weight that everybody can take. And it doesn't cost you any money. In fact, it actually *saves* you money. What could be better than that?

But nature abhors a vacuum, you know. Right now, you're probably asking yourself, "But Bill! If I don't drink sodas and stuff . . . what am I supposed to drink?"

That's an easy one. Instead of drinking processed beverages, I want you to . . .

Fit Tip #2: Start Drinking Water

That's right. Lots and lots of water. Yes, you'll go to the bathroom a lot (I hear this complaint most often). To which I say: fantastic! Each time you use the bathroom, you'll be flushing impurities out of your system. In fact, these additional trips to the bathroom are a necessary stage in your journey to lose weight, get fit, and stay that way. Here's how it works:

Water intake is essential for metabolizing fat. In other words, you won't be able to lose any weight without water to flush out the by-products of fat that your body has broken down. And here's the part that astounds me: *Our bodies are designed to flush out the impurities they've retained longest before getting rid of the new fluids we've just ingested.* Which means that those first few times you're running to the bathroom, you're not just getting rid of excess fluids. You're actually starting a very deep and healthy cleansing process that permeates your whole body.[15]

In other words, you're getting rid of that bacon double cheeseburger you ate a few days back, not to mention the hot dogs you overindulged in at the summer cookout, or the several helpings of tiramisu you kicked yourself for eating at a party. And so on and so on. You get the idea.

All those things would stay in you longer (accumulating, piling on top of each other) if your body didn't flush them out. And to flush them out, you need water, plain and simple.

But water has other proven benefits. For instance:

- Water hydrates the skin, and hydrated skin looks younger. It's also more supple and more wrinkle free. By drinking lots of water, you flush out a lot of the impurities that cause blemishes and cracks, leaving your skin glowing and clean-looking. Not bad, right?

- Drinking lots of water also improves your muscle tone. Our muscle tissue needs to be properly hydrated in order to contract properly. In essence, it doesn't matter how hard or how often you exercise. If your muscles aren't properly hydrated, they start to look flabby. The skin surrounding them starts to sag. Does this sound pleasant? Of course it doesn't. So have a glass of water for your muscles' sake, if nothing else.

- Many chronic ailments (headaches, fatigue, back pain, etc.) can actually be caused by dehydration. It makes sense when you think about it. Consider that our muscles are 75 percent water. Our blood is 82 percent water. Our brains are 76 percent water. Our lungs are 90 percent water. Without enough water, our bodies can't work to their optimum capacity. Our systems weaken, becoming more susceptible to disease.[16]

- Here's one of my favorites: *Drinking lots of water will naturally curb your hunger pangs.* And the less hungry you are, the less you'll snack between meals. And the less you do that, well . . . isn't it clear? You lower your calorie intake and start to lose weight naturally.

Try it. Go on. See for yourself. Have a drink of water on me. Have another, and then another. Go on and drink yourself straight into fitness. What could be simpler than that?

More Bad News from the Diet Industry

But wait! Here's another ploy the diet industry likes to use to get you to buy their products. I call it the One Size Fits All plan. They tell you that the pill or machine or plan or CD or DVD set they're selling will work for everyone! Which simply isn't true.

Remember:

> *Weight management isn't a cookie-cutter system. What works for one person might not work for another. The weight you carry results from a number of highly personal factors. So the way you lose the weight must be highly personal, too. You have to learn what works with your body, your mind, and your motivations.*

In other words, no one product will work for everyone. Beware of diet industry products that intimate that they do. It's a sales gimmick, nothing more. Remember, they don't really understand you, nor do they really care to. They just want your money.

These companies know how badly you want to shed pounds. They also know what fitness studies have indicated for years: Many people who lose weight will eventually put the pounds back on. Up to two-thirds of them will put on *more weight* than they lost.[17]

By the way, this is hardly a secret. According to a 2006 study reported in the *New England Journal of Medicine*:

> *Most people who participate in weight loss programs "regain about one-third of the weight [they] lost during the next year and are typically back to baseline in three to five years."*

Why does this happen? The reasons are clear (we've already started to cover it): Most people's efforts at weight loss don't get built on a lifestyle foundation. They're built on fad diets, energy bars, designer gym clothes, mail order products, the latest workout programs . . . and on and on. In other words:

Most people are trying to buy a silver bullet rather than change something fundamental about themselves! I wanted that silver bullet, but I learned that it doesn't exist.

Most people have tied their level of fitness to a multibillion-dollar American weight loss industry whose sole purpose is to take our money, rather than to train us how to live healthier lives.

Here's what I learned from the staff at Duke:

> *The only way to lose weight and get fit is to take the road less traveled. You have to take a hard look at yourself. You have to identify who you are and the habits you've accumulated—the habits that make us fat. There's a word we'll use to refer to these habits. It's a powerful word and you've heard it before. I've used it once and I'll use it again. It's lifestyle, pure and simple.*

Okay, you're probably saying by now, "I get it, Bill, this lifestyle thing is important. But what does it really mean? Can you tell me in practical terms?"

I think I can. We'll start like this, with Fit Tip #3.

Fit Tip #3: Keep a Food Journal (or "Dear Diary, I Just Ate . . . What?!?")

This is one of the first things we learned at Duke, and one of the most important. I want you to start it immediately. Not tomorrow. Today. It's such a simple little habit that anyone can do it. I want you to write down everything you eat. We'll call this record a food journal.

A food journal works like a master detective. It helps you identify what your current lifestyle is, and how you can start to change it. Keeping a food journal is also one of the most effective ways to lose weight.

It could very well be that you've been taking for granted the food you've been putting into your body. No matter how healthy we think we are, most of us don't pay much attention to what we eat on a day-to-day basis. Until we start keeping a food journal, that is.

I know, I know. You're thinking, *Wait a minute, Bill. This can't be right. You can't lose weight by scribbling notes about what you're eating. The only way to lose weight is to eat all kinds of unsavory rabbit food and jog on a treadmill three hours a day.*

Absolutely wrong. Studies have shown that keeping a food journal can double the amount of weight you lose. That's right. I said *double*. In fact, I read a very interesting study published in the August 2008 issue of the *American Journal for Preventative Medicine*. The study was conducted by the Kaiser Permanente Center for Health Research in Portland, Oregon, and it tracked nearly 1,700 participants who were asked to start a simple fitness regime. As part of the regime, participants had to:

- follow a meal plan that was rich in fruits, vegetables, and low-fat or non-fat dairy

- exercise at moderate intensity levels for at least 30 minutes a day

- keep a food journal

- attend weekly support meetings where their food diaries would be collected and discussed.

Can you guess what kinds of results were achieved? After six months, the average weight loss among the participants was thirteen pounds. And more than two-thirds of the participants—69 percent in fact—lost nine pounds, a very important number. By losing those nine pounds, the participants were judged to have reduced their health risks sufficiently to continue their work in the program's second phase.

But here's the really interesting part: *The participants who kept daily food journals lost twice as much weight as their counterparts who kept no records at all.* In fact, the evidence was so striking that Dr. Jack Hollis, one of the study's lead authors, concluded, "It seems that the simple act of writing down what you eat encourages people to consume fewer calories."[18]

Why does it work? Because *writing down the food you eat forces you to pay attention to it.* Think about it. Suppose you go to a movie. The lights go down. The film reel starts. You're quickly drawn into the story. Then someone hands you a big bag of salted, buttered popcorn. You know deep down it's not good for you, but you're really into the story. So you take a few pieces of popcorn and eat them and stare at the screen, wondering what's going to happen next. An hour or two later, the lights come up and—what's this? The popcorn's gone!

Has this ever happened to you? Of course it has, it's happened to all of us. You ate the popcorn because it was there (number one) and because you were distracted from thinking about how bad it was for you (number two). The definition of distraction is *a state where you aren't paying attention.* Paying attention to what we eat is one of the keys to getting fit.

You still don't believe me? Then consider this: A study released in 2001 detailed how French researchers recruited forty-one women who ranged in age from twenty-six to fifty-five. The women were asked to eat lunch once a week in a laboratory setting, and under varying conditions. As they ate, scientists would monitor them. The various conditions under which the women ate were:

- alone, without any distraction

- alone, but listening to recorded instructions on how to focus on the taste of the foods they were eating for lunch

- alone, while listening to a recorded detective story

Regardless of what condition they found themselves in, the women all reported equal levels of hunger. But can you guess under which condition they ate more food, and therefore took in more calories? Correct. The women ate considerably more while listening to the detective tale.[19]

So there really is something to that bit of advice that you shouldn't eat while watching TV or catching up on that movie you've been waiting to see or chatting with friends on your cell phone and on and on and on. Focusing on what you eat is one of the keys to maintaining a healthy weight, as well as to shedding pounds. And there's no better, simpler tool for focusing on what you eat than writing it down in your food journal.

I can attest to this personally. I'll never forget what I wrote down when I first started keeping my food journal. The first time out, we were asked to jot down what we ate on a typical evening at home. I wrote:

"Extra large fries and a Coke from the drive-through at McDonalds."

Because, as perhaps you'll recall, I liked McDonald's french fries best. But for sandwiches, it was Burger King all the way. So under "Extra large fries and a Coke," I wrote:

"Fried chicken sandwich and a bacon double cheeseburger."

I thought about it a moment, then added:

"Actually, this was my late night snack . . ."

I put my pen down and looked at what I'd written. Frankly, I couldn't believe it. Deep down I knew this sort of eating was bad for me, but it was different seeing it right there in front of my face, scratched down in ink *in my own handwriting*. Somehow it seemed more permanent, more immediate and personal. Which of course is the point.

Another medical doctor, Keith Bachman, is part of the Weight Management Initiative at Kaiser Permanente. Regarding this feeling of personal responsibility, Dr. Bachman says, "It's the process of reflecting on what [we] eat that helps us become aware of our habits, and hopefully changes our behavior." He also noted (helpfully) that "keeping a food diary doesn't have to be a formal thing. Just the act of scribbling down what you eat on a Post-It note, sending yourself e-mails tallying each meal, or sending yourself a text message will suffice."[20]

But in addition to recording *what* you're eating, I want you to write down *why*. You may ask: *Bill, what's the purpose in this?* Simple. Writing down *why* you're eating begins to reveal the mindset you're in when you eat, as well as any emotional triggers that might cause you to overeat.

For instance, in my food journal I tried to record the *why* of eating all that fast food for a late night snack. Invariably, I would write something like, "I wasn't full," "I was still hungry," or "I didn't want to go to bed empty."

Later, in group sessions that I attended at Duke, I began to spot certain emotional states that triggered my unhealthy eating. And then I began to decode what my *whys* really meant in terms of my own psychology. For instance:

- When I wrote down, "I wasn't feeling full," I could translate that to mean *I wasn't feeling fulfilled.*

- When I wrote down, "I was still hungry," that was like saying *I still wanted more* (or *I wasn't fulfilled*).

- When I wrote down "I didn't want to go to bed empty," I was pretty much admitting how empty I felt in the first place.

So let's talk about you and your food journal. Maybe in the *What* column, you'll jot down something like:

"Ate a bag of potato chips."

It would help if you could figure out how many potato chips you ate. Check the bag. Was it one ounce, five ounces, eight ounces, ten? Guesstimate if you have to and try to be accurate. If you ate about half of an eight-ounce bag, write down "four ounces."

Okay, so far so good. Now let's deal with the *Why* column. Maybe in the *Why* section, you write something like:

"Got home from work and wanted to relax."

Huh. That's a pretty powerful statement, right? Essentially you're saying that the way you relax from a hard day's work is to eat. And not just to eat anything—you're eating a bag of potato chips, a deep-fried snack food that's notoriously high in sodium and fat.

I know, I know. I can already hear what you're saying. *But Bill! What if I don't eat the fried potato chips? What if I eat the baked kind, which contain less fat and are healthier for you?*

Believe it or not, I'd say, "Good for you!" Eat the baked kind, that's a great first step. After all, it shows that you're *paying attention* (hint, hint, hint). Take a good look at what you just did. You just used your food journal to:

- identify an eating habit (eating habits are part of your lifestyle)

- identify an unhealthy food you're consuming as part of this habit

This would be great if you stopped right here. But suppose you're the person who just raised a stink about baked chips instead of fried? In that case (again) congratulations. You've already begun your new lifestyle. Meaning that you've already used your food journal to:

- come up with a healthier substitute that will help you begin to lose weight

But why stop there? How cool would it be if you wrote down something like this in your food journal instead:

"Got home from work. Ate an apple to relax."

Because of course apples are even healthier for you than baked potato chips. Better still, I'd love to have you write something like:

"Got home from work and needed to relax so I ate an apple, then went for a quick twenty-minute walk around the neighborhood."

Wow! Now that's impressively fit, a practice that combines a healthier eating habit with a bit of mild exercise. Fantastic!

But let's not get ahead of ourselves. Let's take the whole program one step at a time. In fact, let's go back to the first scenario we talked about, when you wrote down:

"What did I eat? About four ounces of potato chips. Why did I eat it? I got home from work and wanted to relax."

Congratulations on writing this down. Let's talk about what you've accomplished. Specifically, you've gained a clear glimpse into a cause that prompts you to eat (work-related stress), and what you ate to compensate for it (a not-so-healthy food). In other words, you've gotten a clear glimpse into your current lifestyle, or a facet of it, at any rate. Now, to go a bit deeper, you could start to ask yourself a few questions, like:

1. What is it at work that's stressing me out?

2. What can I do to fix it?

Also:

3. Why do I deal with stress by eating in the first place?

The Lifestyle That Was Killing Me

So there I was, sitting in that conference room at Duke, a fat kid in a room full of other people just like me, listening to the speaker summarize the program at the Diet & Fitness Center. And the more she kept talking, the more I began to get the idea that something was fundamentally off in *my understanding of my weight.* It wasn't food that was keeping me fat. My habits were keeping me fat, and being fat was killing me.

I remember looking around the room and thinking, *I'm not alone.* That might have been the first belief to change, and it was a big one. In fact, I think it's fair to say that everyone at the orientation session on my first day at Duke was in the same boat. I'm pretty sure that I was the only person who'd stared at his puffy soccer ball face in the mirror of the men's room of the Pegasus restaurant after deep and searing chest pains sent him reeling away from the bar. But so what? Looking around the room that day, I got the distinct and vivid impression that my classmates had lived through situations that were just as awful. Perhaps even worse. And we'd all come to the same decision. In one way or another, we'd all thought: *I will not live like this anymore. In fact, I declare that this isn't living! I have to change and I have to change now, but to do that, I need some help. And that's why I've chosen to come here.*

The lifestyles my classmates and I had created for ourselves weren't working, but the orientation speaker told us that this was good news. She said that once people figure out that something isn't working, they've already taken the first big step toward changing their behavior. In other words, the very admission that there's a problem places your feet on the road to change. That's a pretty big part of the process, she said. And for you, dear reader, it's probably the reason you picked up this book. You deserve to be applauded for that. It took a lot of guts. Congratulations.

But now comes the sobering news. Placing your feet on the road is good, but now you have to walk. In some cases, you might be shocked to find that *you don't know how to do it!* Real change—true change—often demands that we abandon everything we *think* we know and start from scratch. Even the basics must be relearned. Certainly, that was the case with me.

Remember, my case was pretty extreme. I weighed more than 312 pounds when I went to Duke. I hadn't the slightest notion what healthy eating was all about (I refer you to TwinkieGate). I didn't know how to exercise. In fact, I sometimes caught myself thinking that I wasn't genetically cut out for being athletic. I had myself convinced that some people come out of the womb all buff and tanned with rock-hard shoulders and chiseled abs. And some people come out looking . . . well, like me.

Note what's really going on in that thought process. Instead of focusing on *how I could change*, I was focusing on convincing myself that *there was no way I could change*. You see what I mean about bad habits? They're incredibly insidious.

But the orientation speaker gave us a lot of hope. She told us that the process for change was actually very simple. The program would address four points to modify our lifestyles, and the four points were:

- We would work on nutrition and diet. Basically, we would learn about calories, carbohydrates, fats, and how they affected our bodies. We would take a hard look at what we were eating and learn how to implement healthier meals that would bring our weight into balance.

- We would work on our fitness levels. Specifically, we would learn how to exercise in ways that were enjoyable and good for us. We would also set realistic fitness goals—marks within reach of our capabilities, and that could be adjusted to build strength, balance, and flexibility.

- We would take classes that dealt in behavioral modification. This way we could talk honestly about what food meant to us and the habits we'd developed around it.

- Finally, we would learn to manage any medical conditions we had, a lot of which were quite likely related to any excess weight we were carrying. I was lucky as far as this last point was concerned. When I first went to Duke, I wasn't suffering from diabetes, hypertension, or any other disease related to my weight. But you can bet that a lot of my classmates were, and that's why this last point is very important. You can't build a house on a shaky foundation. You have to make sure that the ground is firm before you can start to work.

It probably sounds pretty simple, right? Just change your lifestyle . . . what's the big deal? Well, if it's so simple, why don't more people do it? Answer: Because it's hard. Changing your old habits and beliefs might be the biggest challenge you'll ever face in your life.

But so what? I did it. And if I did it, so can you. Remember, I'm no one special. I just got really fed up at all the missed opportunities, the endless shame, a horizon that always lay out of reach. I got sick and tired of the life I'd been living. My question right now is: Have you?

And just so we're clear. Forget all the pills. The magic shakes. The celebrity exercise DVDs. This is the hard way, the only way, the way that really works. Lifestyle change is not just for a couple of months. It's for the rest of your life.

And so I began to work on myself. And this is what I did . . .

PART TWO:

FAT KID GETS FIT

My First Week at Duke

The program started the very next morning, Monday at 9 a.m. My classmates and I enjoyed a preselected breakfast in the DFC cafeteria. I mention that it was preselected because later on, as the program progresses, choosing your menu becomes a big part of your training, a very important exercise. But since we were all brand new to the center, they made that first choice for us.

Breakfast that first day consisted of a low-calorie, balanced meal like one of the healthy options I've listed below:

- Breakfast quesadilla—170 calories

- Fruit serving—60 calories

- ½ cup of skim milk—45 calories

Or:

- 1 cup of oatmeal—160 calories

- 6 egg white omelet—90 calories

- Vegetable side—15 calories

Or:

- 2 banana walnut pancakes—215 calories

- 2 tablespoons of strawberry maple syrup—40 calories

- ¼ cup of yogurt—45 calories

Or:

- 1 egg Benedict with hollandaise sauce—275 calories

- ½ cup of skim milk—45 calories

- Fruit serving—60 calories

Or:

- 2 whole wheat blueberry pancakes—180 calories

- 2 tablespoons of light syrup—15 calories

- ¼ cup of cottage cheese—45 calories

- Fruit serving—60 calories

And so on.

I offer these options to show you what breakfast was like that very first day at Duke, as well as to show you what kind of meals you can have on an intake of 1,200 calories per day, which is about what I started off with. Twelve hundred calories might sound pretty low, but it's in the standard range (for men, at least) when you start the DFC program.

After breakfast, we had our physical examinations. This included a full-on stress test called an ETT, or Exercise Tolerance Test. You know the kind I'm talking about. Technicians put you on a treadmill and wire you up to an EKG to check how your heart will react to work. The reason for this exam was that the center wanted to make sure that our bodies were ready for physical exercise. As you might well imagine, some people who first attend the Duke DFC have a very limited capacity for exercise.

The next day, Tuesday, the staff took some blood. Thankfully, all my tests came back fine. My ID badge for the center was stamped with a tag that said CLEARED FOR EXERCISE. I wasn't necessarily shocked by this, but it still felt pretty good. It was the first time I liked anything that resulted from a workout.

When I talk to some people, they sort of assume that being at Duke was like being at boot camp or diet prison or something. I can hear it in their voices whenever they ask me what Duke was like. "When did they wake you up in the morning?" they ask. "How did they treat you? Were you allowed to make phone calls?" That sort of thing.

I always find this really amusing because being at Duke wasn't prison at all. If anything, I was in prison *before* I got to Duke. Duke is the place where I broke out.

Really, the Diet & Fitness Center felt more like going to college. The day was divided up into slots that you filled by selecting classes you were interested in. We went to classes whenever we wanted, but no one stood over us cracking a whip. That would sort of defeat the purpose. The staff kept telling us time and again: They couldn't do the work *for* us; this was something we had to do on our *own*. They were simply there to present us with the facts. This was Duke University. At Duke they don't dabble in magic charms—they study. They teach. They practice science and medicine. Certain skills can be taught, said the staff, and we will teach them to you. What you do with them—that's up to you.

In other words, the program became as aggressive as we wanted it to be. It all depended on what each person brought to the table, nothing more. I crafted a very full program for myself. By which I mean that I made a point to attend every class that I could. I hadn't gone all that way to slack off. I was there to get better. That was my goal. More fit. Less fat. As simple as that.

Each daily slot offered a class that spoke to one of the four groups of improvement our orientation leader had talked about. Classes on nutrition taught us about food—what's healthy and what's not. Classes on physical fitness taught us how to exercise. Classes in behavior put the spotlight on our eating habits and led us to question which ones were healthy, as well as which ones we should change. And so on.

The center's physical fitness classes spoke to three basic categories of wellness: aerobic, strength-building, and flexibility. Aerobic classes included water aerobics and step exercises. Strength classes covered basic weight resistance training and body sculpting; some of these classes were held in the gym and some were held in the pool. The flexibility classes included yoga, t'ai chi, and basic stretching. Basically, there was something for everyone at every time of day. There were also activities that we could take home with us.

The first fitness class I took was water aerobics. Oddly enough, it was the one thing I felt comfortable doing. I say "oddly enough" because, as you may very well recall, I had previously avoided pools so much that I smiled my way through a broken femur, knowing that I wouldn't have to take high school swim class. But Duke was different. Suddenly I felt perfectly comfortable with the idea of putting on a bathing suit. Looking back, I think I know why: I would not be the only person jumping into the pool. There would be many others like me. In fact, everyone else would be like me. By the way, the metaphor of everyone being in the same pool was not lost on me at the time. We were all in it together, battling the same thing.

Water aerobics turned out to be the perfect type of exercise for someone new to working out. Water offers tremendous resistance against even the tiniest movements, and the buoyancy of being in water lessens the impact on muscles and joints. The instructor gave us Styrofoam paddles we pushed through the pool again and again. I was surprised to find how tired I was after forty-five minutes of this.

In classes on stressful eating, we discussed what food meant to us. In those groups, the staff encouraged us to share how we often used food to bolster our spirits even when our emotions were flat, or sinking fast as the case may be. Other classes dealt in self-esteem, which of course is tied to so many things, not the least of which is what we allow ourselves to put into our bodies. Some classes taught us how anger can sometimes be channeled straight into our stomachs. Other classes helped us target our life motivations and restructure our habits so we could build on these motivations in ways that were healthy and positive.

This was the first time in my life that I'd ever felt comfortable talking so openly about my eating habits. Part of this was due to the fact that the staff at Duke was so caring and professional; I can't overstate that enough. But I also felt safe because everyone else in the group was in the same boat that I was.

At one point or another, we'd all used food to buoy our emotions. If I felt sad, I ate. If I felt happy, I ate. Having emotional connections to food is actually a pretty common phenomenon, except that, in our cases, we'd let things get out of control. Our bodies had put on too much weight. We had to readjust. I told the story of TwinkieGate, and listened as my classmates shared some pretty revealing tales of their own. Everyone had their TwinkieGate moment. The details were different, but the essence stayed the same.

My class wasn't the only group at the center during that time. Duke has a rolling admissions process so there were some people in our sessions who'd started the program a few weeks back and were further along in the process. There were also some people who'd gone to the DFC before and were coming back to refresh themselves. This process of intermingling became incredibly important. My classmates and I—the "newbies"—were able to hear from people who had already gone through the program. Many of them had had great success, consistently meeting their goals for years. Hearing how they did that, and the challenges they'd overcome—hearing that somebody *had* gone all the way through and come out fit on the other side—that became an invaluable part of the process for me. A true inspiration.

But maybe one of the most basic shifts that took place for me at Duke was the stark, mathematical view I took of the food I had once put into my body. As I said, the DFC offered plenty of classes that broke down the nutritional elements of food and guided us to look more thoroughly at what we were really consuming.

It would be impossible for me to outline every single class I took, nor would I presume to do so. Like I said, I'm not an expert. But I can say this: Duke chose a basic and common-sense approach to analyzing food intake. To promote developing healthy eating habits, they boiled the whole process down to *calories in versus calories out.*

Do the Math

In the beginning of this book, I said that you won't have to become an expert on nutrition or physiology to get fit the way I did. Please don't misunderstand me—knowledge of these subjects is critical, and I encourage you to read up on them. But a faster, more common-sense approach for getting fit exists, and the best part is, you already know how to do it. Because weight boils down to simple addition and subtraction. For instance:

Let's say you take in 4,000 calories a day and only burn off 2,500. Your body will store the remainder, any remainder (in this case 1,500 calories) as fat. What could be simpler than that?

But suppose you kept this up for a month. That's 1,500 calories a day x 30 = 45,000 calories stored as fat. Hmmm. You might be thinking that's a lot. But hang on a second. We're just getting started.

Suppose you kept up your excess eating for a year. Or two. Or three. I'm sure you're starting to get the point. My classmates and I did, certainly. It soon became painfully clear that most of us had been putting more calories into our bodies than we'd been burning off, and doing so for long periods of time. Year after year. Sometimes for our entire lives.

Now here's something else you should probably know:

One pound of body weight is equal to 3,500 calories. Which means that, in order to lose or gain one pound, you either have to subtract or add 3,500 calories.

So let's go back to our first situation. You take in 4,000 calories a day and only burn off 2,500. Your body stores the remainder, which is 1,500 calories. That's a little less than half a pound. Keep that up for seven days and guess what! You've just stored 10,500 calories, or 3 pounds even.

Now you might be thinking, *Wow! Three pounds?!? Just like that? In a week?!?*

Well, sure. Like I said, there's no mystery to it. It just boils down to math. But that can work both ways, you know. For instance, I just showed you how gaining weight happens by adding calories. But losing weight is basically the same. You can lose weight by reversing the equation. In order to lose weight you must:

Eat less (consume less calories) while burning more off (increase your exercise).

How do you do this? Create a lifestyle where you plan sensible meals and take regular exercise. *Keep that up over time and the weight will come off.* It sounds simple, and it is.

Please note that I said "over time." Proper results do not come overnight, but they do come—that much is certain. You just have to stick to your plan.

Like I said, at the DFC, I was on a regimen of 1,200 calories a day. I know: that may not sound like a lot to you, but I was constantly surprised by *how much* food I was able to eat and still not exceed that amount. Twelve hundred calories can be quite sufficient if you're eating the right kinds of food, by which I mean foods that are low in fat and low in sodium. Follow an educated menu plan and you can really pack the food away and still stay low in calorie count.

Basically, I ate 250 calories for breakfast, another 300 calories for lunch, and 600 calories for dinner. Along with that, I was encouraged to drink at least 64 ounces of fluid per day (or eight 8-ounce glasses). The fluids could be water, of course, but I could also substitute unsweetened lemon drink, herb teas, coffee, some forms of unsweetened fruit punch . . . anything with negligible sodium and calorie counts. Personally, I preferred water and lemon drink, the benefits of which we've already discussed. But I also drank coffee and Crystal Light.

And I was told not to skip any meals! In other words, I was told not to reduce my calorie intake any further than I already had. This may sound like a strange thing to stipulate. You'd probably think that anyone eating 1,200 calories a day would be, if anything, constantly hungry. But it actually makes a whole lot of sense when you consider how badly some people want to lose weight. It's Diet Thinking all the way, and very misguided on so many levels. And yet some people start to figure, "Hey! Wait a minute! If I cut out an extra hundred or two hundred calories a day, I'll lose the weight in a jiff!" Nothing could be more incorrect.

Restricting food intake beyond certain levels only makes a person cranky, desperate, and highly fatigued, to say nothing of the terrific toll it takes on your heart, brain, and other major organs. Besides that, food restriction is symptomatic of a personality that's looking for a quick fix, and we already know what happens to them. They put the weight back on again, usually with a lot to spare, and usually very quickly. Far better to stick to a tried-and-true plan and take things slow and easy. Remember: A diet is fast and immediate—and temporary. A lifestyle is living a balanced, successful, healthy life that also lets pounds fall off.

Now keep in mind exactly where I was coming from. I went from eating 1,600 calories *for breakfast* to a regimen in which I consumed 400 calories *less* than that *throughout the course of an entire day*.

How did that feel? You know what? Not bad! I remember being a little hungry at the end of each day, but it wasn't like an *I'm-famished-this-is-the-end-of-the-world* kind of hungry. In fact, it wasn't very uncomfortable at all. Probably thanks to the exercise I was doing, I was tired by the time each day was over, but not exhausted. More like pleasantly spent. I felt like I'd worked, and was ready for bed.

Once in a while, we would go to the Northgate Mall, which was located right near the center. The staff at the DFC encouraged these trips. "Go walk the mall," they would tell us. Because walking, of course, was good exercise, but also because you could do it with friends and participate in life. The whole point of being at Duke was not to cut yourself out from the world at large, but to build a new life in it. Your life didn't stop when you got to the center. Your life carried on, but with new ideas and a brand new set of skills for living, none of which would have been valuable if we couldn't begin to practice them. Therefore, getting out was a must, and the Northgate Mall was one of those places we went to be part of the world.

So the first few days passed by pretty fast. Some folks started to see results right away, but I sure as heck wasn't one of them. In fact, very soon, I experienced what today I call a . . .

Crisis Point!

had told myself again and again, *I can do this. I am* going *to do this. I am* going *to lose the weight!* And I'd made sure I stayed absolutely 100 percent on the program. I kept my meals to 1,200 calories a day. I exercised. I went to my classes. I learned what the staff at Duke was teaching. When I didn't understand something, I raised my hand and asked questions. I think it's pretty safe to say I was really in swing with the program.

But by the end of my first week, it was clear that I wasn't losing any weight. Our program called for us to step on the scale at the end of each week. And the first time I stepped on the scale my numbers hadn't budged a bit. I was doing everything the Duke staff told me to do, but I still weighed 312 pounds. Talk about a bleak moment. I can't describe how awful that felt, nor can I describe the horror show that started playing out in the theater of my head right then. Insidious, damaging, angry, awful, self-defeating thoughts rose up, creating a kind of cacophony.

How is this possible? I thought. *Wait a minute . . . maybe it* isn't *possible. See? I knew I couldn't do it . . . I told ya, I told ya, I told ya . . .*

This is stupid. What was I thinking? . . .

I'm an idiot. Look at me . . . driving all the way down to North Carolina just to fail. I always knew that I would . . .

And so on.

This was a difficult moment for me. Being fat had always been bad enough. But now I felt terribly certain that I would have to stay fat forever. I couldn't lose weight. I'd tried and I'd failed. That failure would mark me the rest of my life.

Luckily, I chose to make an appointment with the clinic nurse before things got too far out of hand. I told her what was happening (or what *wasn't* happening, more precisely). She said, "Were you doing any outside eating?"

Outside eating meant eating food that hadn't been served by the center. And yes, this was certainly possible. As I've said, during my first time at Duke, I'd taken a room at the hotel/apartment complex directly across the street from the center. Duke wasn't running a penal colony— I was free to come and go as I pleased. I could certainly go to a snack machine and get myself a candy bar, or drive into town and go to a restaurant, a drive-in, or an ice cream shop.

But: "No," I said. I hadn't been eating anything but the food on my plan. So the nurse sent me off to see Dr. Michael Hamilton who, at that time, was the program's director.

Dr. Hamilton is a very kind and patient man. I explained the situation to him and he listened very closely. "Well," he said, and he gave a little shrug. "Usually we do see *some* weight loss after the first week. But not to worry. Just stick with it. Stick to it."

Looking back, I feel pretty certain that the Duke staff had seen a situation like mine before. I also think that, at that point, Dr. Hamilton knew something I myself had never suspected: that human bodies sometimes take a little nudging to fall into new routines. But the biggest danger of all (by far) was that I might start to lose hope.

"But what should I be doing differently?" I said.

Looking back, I can see that this is the classic question for a results-oriented person. If you're not reaching your goal, then change your technique for getting there. Not so, according to Dr. Hamilton.

He shook his head. "Nothing. Don't change a thing. Stick with it, that's all."

So I did, and he was right. When I went back the next week to weigh myself, I had noticeably lost weight. I remember that moment very well. I climbed on the scale and closed my eyes and took a deep breath and let it out, prepared to be disappointed again. But this time the nurse said, "Good. It looks like you're down a few pounds."

I almost couldn't believe it.

I asked the nurse to check it again. She smiled and said, "Nope. Don't worry. It's right. You're down a few pounds. Congratulations."

That's when the dam inside me broke. That's when I looked out the window and saw what a cold and blustery day it was. The sky was dark gray. I don't think I'll ever forget that. I realized that I was in Durham, North Carolina, and I had just done the most miraculous thing I had ever done in my entire adult life. I had just lost weight! However small, however much effort it had taken, I had finally lost some weight!

Now here's the part that I always tell people, and some of them just don't get it. Did I celebrate? Did I dance a jig? Did I get really high on myself? Nope. I didn't. I don't even remember how many pounds I'd lost at that second weigh-in. It wasn't really important to me because I'd been listening to everything we were learning at Duke. And one of the things they teach is that fixating on your weight can be incredibly counterproductive. So I didn't pay much attention to the number. Instead, I put my attention on how much I enjoyed that moment. How determined I was to do it again.

This isn't anything big, I thought. *This is just the new normal.*

I'd decided to lead a new lifestyle, and losing weight and getting fit were a big part of that. Ergo: From that point forward, losing weight would be business as usual. And I promised myself I would keep losing weight until I had reached a place where I felt comfortable.

Not any particular number, you see. Just comfortable. That was all.

Winning by Losing

stuck with water aerobics for the rest of my time at Duke. I played basketball here and there, but nothing too crazy and nothing intense—more like going out on the court with a couple of friends to throw the ball around.

Toward the end of the four-week program, a big part of our education came in the form of what I call the "Experiences." These were real-life exercises designed to help us master the skills that would keep our programs running smoothly as we segued back to our lives in the world that existed outside the center. There was the Grocery Store Tour. The Restaurant Experience. Eating on the Road. In the real world, people shop at a grocery store. They go out to eat at restaurants. They sometimes have to eat on the road. So we needed to know how to do these things as part of our new lifestyle.

The Grocery Store Tour was literally that: Our class went out to a supermarket on a guided field trip. Before that, we'd taken classes on nutrition labels and how to read them, what the stats on the labels mean, and how they apply to healthy eating—or don't, as the case may be. I really enjoyed this part of my education, mostly because I found the Grocery Store Tour to be a pleasantly academic exercise. Once you read a food item's label, you have a certain power over it, specifically the power to choose whether it fits into your plan or not, and therefore whether you'd eat it or not. Nothing is left to guesswork.

Mind you, we didn't go to the store to buy anything. We went to observe how the store was laid out, and specifically to strategize about which foods we *would* buy for ourselves, the ones that led to fitness and health and kept us aligned with our lifestyle plan. Here are some things we learned right off the bat:

- *Never visit a grocery store when you're hungry.* This isn't just an old wives' tale. It's practical, sound advice. Going to a supermarket when you're hungry increases your tendency to buy food on impulse, and often food that's not suitably healthy—food that you'll later regret.

- *Make a list before you go.* Once you're familiar with the foods you like to eat to stay within your lifestyle, write them down on a list. Better yet, use your list as a menu plan for a week's worth of menus, possibly two. Making a list is very important since lists can be checked with your brain instead of your stomach. And of course making a list also decreases your tendency to impulse shop. Think of it like a set of rules. You've tested the rules. You know that they work. That's why you choose to stick to them.

- *Don't wander around the aisles.* Shopping for food is a household task, like mowing the lawn or doing the laundry. There's no need to rush, but don't linger either. Do it briskly. Do it with energy. Take your list. Get what you need, then get out.

- *Stay away from (some) processed foods.* This is a very important rule, and one that gains even more importance as more and more of the foods we eat endure some kind of treatment. Processing isn't necessarily healthy. Why not? Good question. Read my next Fit Tip.

Fit Tip #4: Stay Away from (Some) Processed Foods

Before we delve too deeply into this, let's establish a vocabulary. By processed foods, I'm referring to any food that's in some way been altered from its original state. As you can imagine, that covers a great deal of food you'll find in our grocery stores. But don't take my word for it. Try it sometime.

Go to your local supermarket and take a Grocery Store Tour of your own. Ask yourself how many foods you see that have been frozen, dehydrated, bleached, canned, fortified, and so forth. Pick up a random container and check the label. Specifically check the level of sodium present, as well as the levels of trans fats and saturated fats. Check the calorie count. Some processed foods will astound you with how high these levels can rise.

Are all processed foods unhealthy? No, not at all. That's why I say "avoid (some) processed foods." Take the case of frozen vegetables, for instance. They're very healthy for you. Freezing is a process used to extend the life of a sack of green beans, cauliflower, or carrots. Fresh vegetables are best, of course, but freezing is probably *second best*. Freezing a vegetable seals in all its essential vitamins and minerals. The freezing process allows you to keep vegetables in your home and enjoy them many months after they normally would have spoiled. So freezing, as a process, is pretty harmless all in all.

Milk is another good example of a processed food that's good for you. Pasteurization and homogenization are two important processes that are commonly applied to milk. Respectively, these processes lower harmful bacteria count and keep fat levels from separating, making the milk we drink more palatable. There are some who claim that milk is more beneficial and nutritious when you drink it completely unprocessed. With respect to people who think this way, I'd have to say that—however you slice it—processed milk is hardly damaging to human bodies.

Okay, that's the good news. Now for the bad.

Other processed foods can throw an absolute monkey wrench in your new quest to stay fit. Take flour and rice for instance, both of which come in bleached varieties that are white and supposedly more palatable. Everyone loves fluffy white rice, don't they? Maybe so. But the bleaching process strips the vital nutrients from the grain. It pulls out the fiber, which is one of the primary reasons flour and rice are so important to eat in the first place.

Little-known fact: Human bodies metabolize bleached flour and rice the same way they would quantities of sugar. In other words, when we eat bleached flour and rice, our bodies give quick rushes of energy instead of long, extended burns. There's really no significant health benefit to consuming processed grains. This includes breads and pastas that are made with processed grains, as well.

Now take a look at canned foods. Most people don't know it, but an essential part of the canning process involves heating the canned food *in the can* to destroy any harmful bacteria that might want to set up shop in there and grow to their hearts' content. Apart from altering the food's texture, the heating process also strips out all the essential vitamins and minerals (sound familiar?). Many canners also add brine—essentially salt water—to protect against pest infestations, and this equates to higher sodium levels, which in turn leads to high blood pressure and heart disease. Sometimes canned goods manufacturers also add oils to season the food, and oils are fattening. Some manufacturers add sugar syrups (especially in the case of canned fruit), which raises the food's sugar content to astronomical heights.[21]

Again, you have to ask yourself: Is this kind of food in line with the lifestyle goals I've set for myself? Once in a while, sure. Why not? But day in, day out? You'll probably find that fresh is the way to go.

Now think of all the packaged snack foods a grocery store typically offers. Go look at the labels on chips and cookies and cakes and cheese treats and the boxes of sugary cereals that so many kids in America eat (and a whole lot of adults, too). Read the labels carefully. Check the calorie content. Check the sodium content. Check the total carbohydrates. Don't fall prey to mitigating claims like "Fortified with Vitamin C!" Trust me, there are better ways to get our vitamin C than through fortification processes. In fact, I'm pretty willing to bet that, once you've read a bunch of these labels, you'll start to look for healthier substitutes—foods that make you fit.

But really the worst offenders in the category of processed foods are the processed meats. Hot dogs. Lunch meats. Sausages. They're high in sodium (shockingly high!). They carry a lot of fats and worse—some of them carry trans fats, the consumption of which increases our risk of coronary heart disease. And studies have shown that eating processed meats in general raises our risk for certain types of cancer, chiefly: kidney, stomach, and colorectal cancer. That's three too many, if you ask me.

Look, I'm not trying to say that you should never eat a hot dog again. I'm not trying to say you should utterly swear off eating a can of nice hot tomato soup the next time winter rolls around and temperatures start to plummet. But I *am* saying this: You deserve information. If you want to get fit, you should know the risks. Do your research. Plan your menus.

Don't think of this as eliminating something you've always really enjoyed. Buy the foods that work with the lifestyle you've chosen to help you reach your goals.

Living a healthy lifestyle means taking a balanced approach to eating. So yes, enjoy your tomato soup. But make sure you're also eating plenty of fresh grains. Make sure you're getting lots of fresh fruits and vegetables. In other words, if you must eat processed foods, don't overindulge. Make sure that you're covering all the bases, then come back to healthier foods.

TwinkieGate Reexplored

The Grocery Store Tour turned out to be one of the most shocking revelations during my time at Duke. Once I'd learned to read a nutrition label, I found it positively astounding to walk through a supermarket, pick up an item I'd always eaten, and see what it really contained. I can't tell you how many labels I read that made me cringe. *Wow, I* thought. *I've been eating that for years! What the heck was I thinking?*

For instance, nothing resonated with me more memorably than when I picked up a pack of Twinkies, flipped it over, and read the label. Here are the nutrition facts:

Nutritional Information for 1 Twinkie

Calories	150
Calories from Fat	40
Total Fat	7% of daily value
Cholesterol	20 mg or 7% of daily value
Sodium	220 mg or 9% of daily value

You might be thinking, *Well, so what? That doesn't sound so bad . . .*
Maybe. But then again, maybe not.

Now it's time for a trivia question. Do you think most kids would open a package of Twinkies and eat just one? I know this fat kid didn't. So, let's double the information above. That brings our total nutritional information to:

Nutritional Information for 2 Twinkies

Calories	300
Calories from Fat	80
Total Fat	14% of daily value
Cholesterol	40 mg or 14% of daily value
Sodium	440 mg or 18% of daily value

Aha, you might be thinking now. One little treat gave me one quarter of my total calorie intake for the day (assuming that I'm sticking to my initial Duke DFC 1,200 calorie count). This treat was also high in fat, and painfully high in sodium.

Worth it? Kids would say that it is, but when I was a kid, I didn't care so much about balancing nutritional needs. I cared about what tasted good. That's why some kids get fat, and that's why some fat kids become fat adults. But this can be fixed. You just have to find a place to start and take it one day at a time.

Again, I'm not saying you can never eat a Twinkie again. The lesson is you can eat a Twinkie as part of a greater plan.

Like I said, I found the Grocery Store Tour tremendously enlightening. But no more so than the Restaurant Experience, where I learned a vital lesson that I now pass on to you. And that lesson is:

Fit Tip #5: When Eating Out, Ask and You Will Receive

For the Restaurant Experience, we literally left the DFC and went out on the town. Duke made us a reservation at the Angus Barn, a steakhouse. But before we went, we met as a class to discuss what we expected to find on our field trip, the challenges we thought might arise. During this session, we read the Angus Barn's menu together and strategized about how to create a meal that would satisfy our goals and make us feel comfortable.

When it comes to eating out, there are literally dozens of tips you can use to stick to your lifestyle. The first thing you need to know is that some restaurants are better than others for people who watch what they eat. And believe it or not, steakhouses are some of the best places you can go. This may sound a bit strange until you stop to consider a few things.

For one thing, every steakhouse I've ever visited has a grilled chicken or fish selection. Order this instead of the higher-fat, cholesterol-laden beef. You can always ask for a dry baked potato. Skip the sour cream they may offer, and who says you have to have butter? By the way, who says you have to eat the whole thing? Cut your potato in half and send half back. Remember: you're in charge of what you eat. You and nobody else.

Another great thing about steakhouses is that they always have fresh-sliced tomatoes and plenty of vegetable sides. Take advantage of this! Ask for half a tomato thinly sliced and placed in a bowl. Ask for a side of spinach, but without the butter or oil. Ask for a small green salad without any croutons and with the dressing on the side. Or better yet, don't use dressing at all. Avoid the oil and fats they carry and treat yourself to a nice complement of balsamic vinegar, one of my favorites! If they bring a basket of bread to the table, ask them to take it away. Bread can really pack on the carbs, and you're watching those, remember?

These days, friends laugh at me because I eat grilled salmon and steamed broccoli at nearly every steakhouse I go to. Why not? It's a healthy, delicious choice. And then there's the company, which is always my real reason for going out in the first place. Some of the greatest, smartest conversations I've ever had have been in restaurants. That's what I'm there for most of all, the fellowship. The experience.

Now compare the facility you might have at a steakhouse to the restrictions imposed by many ethnic restaurants. I love Indian food, but I find it hard to eat in an Indian restaurant because (very often) so much of the food is already prepared with heavy fat. That's always been a bit of a sacrifice for me (I really, *really* love Indian food!). But I'm willing to sacrifice here and there to stay in touch with my long-term goals.

Another grand misconception I hear from time to time is that there's no way anyone can eat healthy at a Chinese restaurant. This is absolutely wrong. Order the steamed mixed vegetables and make sure to ask for a side of the low-sodium soy sauce. Yes, you should stay away from anything breaded and deep-fried, but really, so what? That still leaves you half the menu, full of delicious entrees. Order the stir-fried vegetables with tofu. Yes, you can eat that, stir-fry is fine, just ask them to use very little or no oil. Generally, the chef will accommodate you. And while we're on the subject, ask the chef to prepare your entree without MSG, which is monosodium glutamate. Lately this food additive—quite typical in modern Asian-style cooking—has been linked to some alarming health problems such as migraines, child hyperactivity, food allergies, neural disorders, and, yes (of course), obesity. But not to worry. Your food won't contain any MSG if you order a nice big bowl of steamed broccoli and snow peas, and a side of steamed brown rice.

Aha! We're back to rice again. Why do I specify *brown* rice? Because brown rice is white rice that hasn't been bleached to make it look cleaner and fluffier. As I've already mentioned, the bleaching process that makes rice white removes a lot of essential nutrients like fiber, zinc, magnesium, and manganese. Brown rice is considered a whole grain. White rice is not. So stick with the brown rice. It's better for you, and every Chinese restaurant I've ever been in has it.

I ended up enjoying my time at Angus Barn very much. The thing I enjoyed most was learning firsthand that going to a restaurant does not have to break your calorie bank. You can go out with friends and family and for business meetings and eat and relax just like everyone else. In fact, that's the biggest lesson the Restaurant Experience taught me, one which I gladly pass on to you:

Going to a restaurant isn't really about the food. It's more about the company you're with, the memories you create, the reason you're there. Now that's a Restaurant Experience, indeed!

Leaving Duke

I stayed at Duke for four full weeks. And during that time, I lost fourteen pounds. In some ways, it seemed like nothing for a guy who'd started out at 312. Losing fourteen pounds isn't really noticeable when you weigh as much as I did, but I'll tell you this: I could *feel* the difference, and that was the most important thing. I'd applied myself to getting healthier and was starting to see results.

I believed in what I had learned at Duke. My instructors had made their lessons clear. I also had the support and well wishes of newfound friends to consider. I vowed that I would stick with my new lifestyle. In fact, I told myself that I had to. In a very real way, my life depended on it. I refused to face another afternoon like the one I'd spent at the Meadowlands in the men's room of the Pegasus Restaurant. Going to Duke had been like crossing the Rubicon. I was never going back to my old ways again. I was on the road to change for good.

Was I nervous to leave the center? Absolutely. No question about it. In fact I was very, *very* nervous, as most people are their first time around. I knew that, outside the DFC, I wouldn't be functioning in an environment that was as supportive as I'd become accustomed to. I'd be leaning more heavily on the skills that I'd learned, and hoping that they would hold me up.

Duke knows that resuming your life can be hard when you leave the center. But I was amazed at the foresight they had in preparing me for my return to the world. For instance, they strongly advised me to reset my daily calorie goal to 1,500. This wasn't some kind of concession, they were simply being realistic. The Diet & Fitness Center has perfected the art of preparing healthy meals. I bet there isn't a kitchen in the country that can pack as much food as they can into a 1,200-calorie daily allow-ance. A 1,500-calorie allowance, when combined with adequate exercise, would still move me toward my fitness goals. My 300 "extra" calories would compensate for my lack of Duke's expertise in the kitchen. This is what my instructors told me, and I have to admit—it struck me as totally logical. But I can't say it put me at ease. I was edgy enough about leaving the center without having to worry about taking on more calories.

However, I decided I had put my trust in Duke for everything else so far. There was no reason to suddenly pull up stakes and stop. I had witnessed firsthand how their reputation and experience could be lever-aged to help me get fit. At fourteen pounds lighter, I also knew that the program they touted was working. So I put aside my worries and fears as best I could and stuck to my routine.

The DFC offered a class called Life After the Center, which focused on how to integrate our new skill set into our lives once we got back home. I took a lot of notes in that class. I wanted to be prepared.

As it turned out, I got to use those skills right away. In fact, I got to use them almost before I'd left North Carolina.

Picture me driving up Route 85 and swinging off the highway into a rest stop. Can you guess which restaurant I visited first after leaving the DFC? Yup. You got it. McDonald's. That's right. And this time, you know what I ordered there? Coffee, and that was all.

I'll never forget this experience. I went through the drive-through and rolled down my window. The voice of the woman manning the inter-com box sounded tinny, like she was talking through a long line of soup cans strung together to make a crude sort of megaphone. "One coffee," she said. "Any cream with that?"

"No cream," I said. "Just coffee."

"How many sugars?"

"No sugars," I said. "Just the coffee, thanks."

She seemed to be asking if I wanted anything else. "A biscuit maybe? Egg McMuffin? Hash browns? Pancakes?" The tone of her voice spoke vol-umes. It was like she was saying, *Ya know. How about ordering some* food?

But again I said, "No thanks. I'm good. Already grabbed something." Which was true.

That morning, just before leaving the center, I'd had a nice bowl of oatmeal with raisins on top and an egg-white omelet. In short, I was full and feeling good. I was ready to keep to my healthy lifestyle.

I knew that I had a long drive ahead. When you're traveling, it seems like every restaurant's just begging you to buy what I like to call . . . well, road food. I think you know what I'm talking about. The burgers. The pizza. The double orders of fries. Basically, everything that made me fat in the first place.

But you know what? Let's be honest. That's not really being fair. The restaurants on highways clear across our country have all gotten the message, more or less. They offer healthier choices now. They were offering healthy choices back then.

Back when I was going through my midnight fast food binging phase while working on the campaign, I could have ordered a salad topped with slices of skinless chicken breast, no dressing. Truthfully, I could have ordered the same salad without the chicken breast, if I'd wanted. No one was twisting my arm to load up the Thousand Island dressing. Nobody was telling me I had to order that bacon double cheeseburger with a super-sized carton of french fries after midnight.

The forces that pushed me to do these things had nothing to do with the restaurants themselves. They had to do with me. Duke showed me that. Once the staff at the center explained it, I saw it all, clear as a bell. I was the one responsible. I was the one in charge. And therefore I could change.

The woman on the drive-through intercom sounded a little confused when I told her I didn't need anything to eat. But she told me the total amount of my purchase and said, "Thank you for coming to McDonald's. Please drive around to the window."

I remember putting my car in gear and thinking about my last visit to the Golden Arches, that big breakfast I'd wolfed down on the same day I checked into Duke. And I knew it had only been a month or so since then, but something had changed. I could already feel it: the feeling of finally knowing there was a path I could take, a road I could walk. It wasn't just fourteen pounds of difference—it went deeper than that. *I was different.*

I was in control of my eating and weight for the very first time in my life. And that, I have to tell you, was a very good feeling, indeed.

My First Gym

I had to keep up my exercise once I'd left the DFC. I had to follow through with the lessons I'd learned, the techniques I'd been taught. But now I was back in my hometown again. It was December—too cold to go for a run outside, or even a walk. And I started to wonder, "Where can I go? I have to go somewhere to work up a sweat."

The folks at Duke had told us how important it was to join a gym, so I set out to find one at home.

There were plenty of options to choose from. My hometown of Hamilton, New Jersey, is full of gyms. But at Duke I'd been surrounded by other people like me, people who were battling their weight. We didn't judge each other; we were all in the same boat, which gave us a certain camaraderie. I quickly learned that this wasn't the atmosphere some gyms liked to promote.

Sometimes a double standard exists when it comes to fat people and gyms. Fit people often look at a fat person and think, *Man, he should go work out or something.* But the moment a fat person shows up at the gym, these same fit people think, *Whoa! What the hell is* he *doing here?!?* You can see it written all over their faces, or the way they try not to stare.

To say the least, I was feeling a little self-conscious about going to purchase a gym membership. So I asked my friend Julie McCord Bethke to go with me while I went to tour a popular facility a few miles from my house. I walked through the door of the place—all 298 pounds of me—and went right up to the woman behind the counter and smiled and asked about joining her gym.

I'll never forget the look she gave me. She was clearly surprised by my request and she frowned at me like I'd done something wrong. Like

I was an idiot. "C'mon. I'll give you the tour," she said. Like the entire procedure was tantamount to having a tooth pulled without anesthesia.

This woman (who was very fit) took off at a lightning-fast pace that clearly seemed designed to discourage me from setting foot in the hallowed halls of this Exercise Sanctum Sanctorum. She speed-walked up and down hallways and around corners. She seemed completely disconnected from me and what I might need. I guess she saw some fat guy who, for some ridiculous reason, had decided to strain the limits of plausibility and kid himself about joining a gym. Her attitude made it very clear that her sole motivation for showing me around was to *get it over with as fast as possible*. Here are the treadmills, there are the weights, and over there are the lockers. Rattling off the words like an auctioneer who was pressing a bid. I'm not even sure she paused to breathe, it was quick quick quick and rush rush rush! Just sprint through the tour and act condescending and fat guy would be gone.

In every room we visited, in-shape, muscular people stopped doing their leg curls and pull downs at the universal machines. Discussions over the relative merits of creatine supplements ground to a halt. Jokes died before the punch line was given. Everyone stared at me. The people working out at this place all looked like models from major clothing catalogs. They were all gorgeous, all of them had zero-point-zero percent body fat, and now every single one of them was gawking at me with obvious distaste. A few even openly snickered.

Touring that gym was not the most inspiring moment of my life, let me tell you. But when the tour was finished, I pulled out my wallet and said that I wanted to join. I don't know who was more surprised—me, my friend Julie, or the lady who'd given us the tour.

I told myself that I didn't care how uncomfortable that place made me. I'd just spent twenty-two years being uncomfortable in my own skin. No other place would ever compare. And anyway, who cares about a little discomfort? I wasn't joining that gym to make friends; I just wanted to use the exercise equipment. I just wanted to get fit, that was all that mattered to me—or, like I said, that's what I told myself. And so, ignoring that little voice inside me (call that voice "Better Judgment"), I filled out the forms and picked up a pen and got ready to sign on the dotted line.

But that's when some instinct took hold of me, the same instinct that would later serve me well as a lawyer. I looked at the woman who'd given the tour—the woman who was now staring at me, clearly praying I would reconsider and bolt for the door and never come back—and I asked her, "Is there a cancellation window?"

The woman behind the counter told me (with a bit of relief in her voice, I thought) that yes, if I wanted to, I was certainly welcome to cancel within a few days. I thanked her and signed my contracts and that was that. I had joined a gym.

Julie and I walked back out to the parking lot. Neither of us said a word. I think we were probably both thinking the same thing: that I'd made a huge mistake—one that was nobly inspired, perhaps, but a huge mistake just the same.

We got into my car and I pulled out of the parking lot and started driving down the street. We hadn't gone more than a mile when we passed the local YMCA. A very strong hunch took hold of me then. I hit my turn signal, waited for traffic, then turned off the road and went into the parking lot.

Julie said, "Where are we going?"

I said, "I just want to check in here, okay?"

We walked inside the Y and approached the reception desk. The woman sitting behind the counter looked, well . . . kind of like me. She looked up and put her book down and smiled. "Hey!" she said. "How you doing today?"

"Pretty good," I said. It was tough not to smile. She had that kind of energy. I said, "I was wondering, I mean, I was sort of thinking about maybe joining a gym—"

"Sure!" she said. She popped up out of her chair and came around her desk. She introduced herself and shook hands. Then she looped one hand through Julie's arm and her other hand through mine as if she'd

known us for years and offered to show us the place like she'd been waiting for us to arrive all day.

Well. She showed us the place, all right. I noticed that the workout
area wasn't as big as the one in the first gym had been. The machines
weren't as modern. But the people! I couldn't believe it. Everywhere I
looked, I saw fat people, thin people, old people, young people, kids,
families, you name it. Everyone.

I felt instantly comfortable. Here was a place where I felt at home. At
a gym! Who would have guessed?

We went back to the desk and I filled out the forms and signed on
the dotted line. No hesitation this time. I remember how Julie cocked an
eyebrow, but I think she knew what I was up to. I thanked the woman
who gave us the tour. Then Julie and I walked back to my car and got
back in and I drove back to the first gym.

Julie said, "You're crazy."

I knew what she meant, but I felt like I had to take control of the
situation. And it seemed very clear to me that a gym where I didn't feel
comfortable couldn't possibly be the gym where I went to fulfill my goals.
I needed someplace I really enjoyed, someplace where I felt welcomed,
not judged. And that meant the Hamilton Y.

The woman who'd signed me up at the first gym was surprised to see
me. It seemed like she tried to hide her relief when I told her I wanted to
cancel my membership, which was less than an hour old. She helped me
fill out the paperwork. Never tried to dissuade me. Actually, now that I
think of it, my quitting so fast may have set some kind of record.

Now let me be clear about this story I've just told you: I know that
the first gym I visited would make a great place for lots of people. It
might make a great place for you. Selecting a gym *must* be a highly personal choice, so my rule of thumb is this: *Find a place that gives you
incentive, one that drives you to go there again and again and look forward
to your workout.* For some people, that'll be a place like the first gym I
mentioned. For me, it was the warm embrace of the local Y.

I started going to the Y the next morning. And I kept going every morning of every day. That became my new routine. And gradually, more pounds came off. And then a few more. And then a few more. Which leads me to my next Fit Tip.

Fit Tip #6: Join a Gym

Go on. Just do it. It isn't hard. Find a place that you like. Make sure it's a place that you can afford. Go inside and introduce yourself to the person behind the front desk. Tell them that you're looking for a place to exercise.

Take the gym's orientation. Let them show you all the machines, the facilities, the classes. Take note of where the locker rooms are and where you can find a scale, since you'll probably end up checking that once a week or so (gyms usually keep the scale in the locker room).

In general, find a place where you feel you'll be comfortable coming in nearly every day. Because if you *are* comfortable, then you *will* want to go in every day.

Okay. Have you got all that? Great. You're on your way. Now let's talk about what you'll do, the way you're going to start working out. Don't worry if you have no experience with exercise. It doesn't matter if you've never picked up a weight before or used a machine. The way we're going to start is actually much simpler than that. You're going to walk.

Simple, right? Just walk. That's it. That's all I want you to do. Go to a treadmill (any gym you join will have a few, I'm sure). Get on it. Set the treadmill for an even pace and go. If the gym has a TV, watch the news or your favorite sitcom. If they don't have a TV or you don't like watching TV, bring a book to read, or a magazine. Sometimes I like to put on headphones and zone out with my favorite music. Whatever you want. It's up to you. This is your time. Make it your own.

Time to hit this point hard: There's no mysterious science to getting fit. Losing weight is really a matter of eating better and less, while working out more. Going to the gym fulfills the exercise portion of your lifestyle, so start going, even if that means you're only there for thirty minutes. A thirty-minute trip to the gym is certainly better than nothing. More important, however, is the fact that you're getting used to the place, the rhythm of it. The energy. You're bound to meet other people at your gym and I want you to say hi to them. This, too, is a very important point.

Think of it like this: Going to the gym is a whole lot more than a mechanical routine. It's more than getting on a treadmill or using the weights and watching the clock tick by. *A big part of any gym's importance lies in meeting and associating with other people who are trying to meet their fitness goals. It lies in participating in a culture of health.*

I've made dozens of friends simply because we happen to work out at the same gym at about the same time every day. Some of these friends are there to lose a few pounds. Some of them are preparing for an Iron Man triathlon. Their specific goals aren't the point. The point is this: By being in their company, being a part of this culture of health, you're not sitting in a fast food restaurant. You're not letting your commitment to yourself slide. You're getting out there. Getting active. And that makes all the difference.

In fact, it makes so *much* of a difference, I think it's time that we discussed:

Fit Tip #7: Look for Nontraditional Gyms

Gyms can be found in surprising places. These days, you don't have to limit your search to traditional workout clubs. In fact, facilities that correspond to the new models of service very often offer services and equipment that are more aligned with first time fitness seekers.

For instance:

- Have you investigated your **local community center**? Lots of cities and towns have one—places like the local Y, a church gym, or a club house. The fees for these places are often quite small, and I urge you to check them out. They might not have state-of-the art equipment, but who cares? People were lifting heavy objects long before they invented dumbbells, right? Your local community center gym is the first place to go for a solid, low-cost exercise experience. As a bonus, you get to meet your neighbors. That's a win-win situation.

- Lately, a new model of exercise facility has started to pop up. They're often called **health and wellness centers**, though sometimes I hear them called health and wellness malls. These places follow a template that's very similar to the Duke DFC. You can think of them as gyms that are tied directly to hospitals, or perhaps a university medical center. And because of this, they provide a much broader and deeper range of health-related services. And these services often help you form a more rounded, holistic approach to your lifestyle.

  So what will you find at a health and wellness center? They have all the usual gym equipment: weights, machines, treadmills, and so on. And yes, you'll find various classes taught like yoga, t'ai chi, spinning, dance, aerobics, meditation, and so on. But there might also be a physical rehabilitation wing right on the premises, a place people go to recover from injuries and surgeries. The center might also offer therapeutic massage services. Or classes in healthy cooking. Nutrition. CPR. Substance abuse recovery. Coping with loved ones with Alzheimer's. Living with diabetes.

  There might be a healthy cafe on the grounds. A juice bar. A spa. A conference center allied with a nearby hotel. Some health and wellness centers offer daycare. Babysitting. Guest speakers. Blood tests. Classes in swimming and lifeguarding.

  Are you getting the picture? Like I said, *these places embrace a total fitness model.* It's one of the reasons I recommend health and wellness centers so highly. Given the wide range of services offered, *health and wellness centers make especially suitable places for people who are just starting out on their fitness journey, or have special needs.* To me, that includes people who have never exercised before. But it also includes people who are dealing with or recovering from a serious health issue, like a heart problem or recovery from an illness.

In my hometown, we have the Robert Wood Johnson University Hospital at Hamilton Center for Health and Wellness. It's an amazing facility filled with dedicated people, and an excellent resource for anyone looking to get fit and stay that way. So check your local hospital or university and see if they offer this kind of service.

Now let's address the expense of joining a gym. Because there's another reason why I call this Fit Tip "Look for Nontraditional Gyms." If you think you can't afford a gym, you might be surprised to find that you have the means to afford one already. Or you simply might need to change your perspective a bit to realize how a gym fits with the new life template you're creating for yourself. For instance:

- Have you looked at **joining a gym as if it's an investment?** It is, you know—you're investing in *you*: your health, your body, your life. The return on this investment is huge, too big to describe in fiscal terms. Sometimes viewing the problem like this can break down any barriers you have and motivate you to juggle some funds, committing them toward your health.

- Or have you considered how you might **combine fitness goals to generate extra income?** By which I mean, have you investigated the economics of the choices you're currently making with an eye toward reallocating resources toward fitness goals?

I'll give you an example. Let's say that you order out for lunch pretty much every day. How much money would you save if you stopped ordering out, made your own lunch at home and brought that to work instead?

As we'll cover a little later on, a big part of Duke's training encouraged us to brown bag our lunches. Remember when that used to be in vogue? You plan your meals at the beginning of the week, buy all the necessary ingredients to make really healthy sandwiches like turkey breast on whole wheat bread with some mustard, lettuce, and tomato. Wrap that up and stick it in a brown paper sack along with an apple or a banana and maybe some sliced carrots or cucumbers. And voila! You have a healthy lunch—one that puts you in charge of what you eat, that lets you easily hit your calorie goals, and saves you a tremendous amount of money!

How much money? I bet you'd be amazed. Sixty, seventy, eighty bucks a month? I doubt that's out of the question.

Coincidentally, that's about the same amount of money you'd pay for dues at a really nice gym. So what are you waiting for? Be kind to your body at the same time you're being kind to your wallet. Take control of what you eat.

By the way, you can certainly extend this concept beyond the model for eating out. For instance, imagine the money you would save if you gave up one or two little food vices here and there. Cupcakes and candy bars, for instance. Or what if it wasn't a food vice at all, but something else that's good for your body. What if you quit smoking, for instance? Cigarettes are expensive, right? Plus, quitting smoking does immeasurable good for your overall state of health. Remember that getting fit isn't just about eating right and starting a program of regular exercise. You might have to examine a lot of other lifelong habits as well.

Here's the idea once again: You can take great strides toward your fitness goals by moving away from bad food and bad habits and putting the money you used to spend on those things toward a new, healthy lifestyle.

But if, for some reason, you still can't get to a gym, don't worry. There are plenty of easy, simple alternatives you can resort to. Let's take a look at a few.

Do you own a bike? Great. Get on it and ride it around the block. Do the same thing tomorrow. Do it again the day after that. Work your way up to two blocks, then three, then four, then five, and so on.

What's that you say? You have a bike, but it's old and needs some care? Not a problem. Find that old bike in the basement, blow the dust off, and check the tires. Oil the chain. You're burning calories doing that. And once you're done, you're ready to go out riding, which will help you burn a few more. Make sure you wear a helmet!

Or how about this: Go for a ten-minute walk after lunch. Or go in the morning, if mornings work better. Or go in the evening. Whatever works. The time doesn't matter. Just walk. Next week, raise your ten-minute target to twelve. Then fifteen. Twenty. Thirty. Thirty-five. Forty. You get the idea? I bet that you do. *There's no good excuse not to start getting fit.*

I know of someone who's stayed fit for years, and during those years, he would go to a gym. But then, to save money, he cancelled his gym membership, went to his local sporting goods store, and bought himself a jump rope. Now he jumps rope almost every day. Sometimes he breaks that up with long walks near his home. He does sit-ups and pushups in his bedroom because you really only need a floor to do sit-ups and pushups. They're classic exercises, great for strength training and balance, and you can schedule them into your day whenever you find the time. Another good thing? They don't cost a penny.

In fact, while we're on the subject, let me point this out: *The exercises I've mentioned above are perfect for when you're traveling.* I often hear people complain that it's tough to stay in shape when they travel. But push-ups and sit-ups? Jumping rope? These are such basic exercises that you can do them practically anywhere, in any country or any hotel, anywhere you go that isn't equipped with traditional exercise facilities. And they're powerful, meaning you can get a great workout from them. Remember this next time you're on the road.

Okay, by now, you're starting to get the point. *Going to the gym is a great way to kick off a healthy lifestyle. But remember, there are lots of different kinds of gyms. If your excuse for not exercising is that you can't join a gym (for whatever reason) . . . stop making excuses!* Get on out and start walking, running, swimming, or riding your bike. Get active! That's what's most important. Fitness follows activity.

So let's say you've found a place that you like to go and work out. Let's say you've taken the plunge and gotten a membership to a gym, a health and wellness center, or your local YMCA. Now I want you to start to consider my next Fit Tip, which is:

Fit Tip #8: Use All Aspects of the Facility

When I first started working out at a gym after leaving Duke, I stuck to taking walks on the treadmill. Nothing fancy, just simple exercise.

Why did I use the treadmill? Because I like to read the paper and I like to watch the news. And I found out I could do both of these things while walking on a treadmill.

This was a great way to start because it kept me motivated. But now that I look back, I see that there were so many other exercises I could have chosen at the local Y I had joined. Which is why I advise you to *get to know the facility you've chosen.* Ask questions. And (as I mentioned before) here's a good rule of thumb: Take your facility's orientation.

In other words, I'm encouraging you to take advantage of the entire facility. Don't get locked into any one routine. I'll explain why in a moment.

By taking an orientation session, you learn where all of the treadmills are, but also the free weights, the pool (if there is one), the classes, the locker rooms, studios. Everything. Why is this important? Part of it has to do with getting comfortable with the space. You want to know where things are located so you can get to them when you need them. But more importantly, you want to see and understand the scope of what's available to you. That way, you'll start to appreciate the variety of activities you can enjoy. You'll also see other people enjoying them, which might make you want to give them a try.

For instance, if you've never been on an elliptical machine before, it could be a little intimidating. At first glance, they might look pretty strange. Your feet move in orbits instead of in steps. The arm poles work in time with the feet, almost as if you are cross-country skiing. And then there are all the buttons and readouts on the console. Who wants to have to deal with all that?

I guess what I'm trying to say is that, if you're shy, it might take you a little while to climb up on an elliptical machine and try it out (I know it took years before I did, but now I *love* the elliptical). But what a shame not to try these machines! Why? Because they can be great for our health. Elliptical machines allow us to get in a great cardiovascular workout at any grade of difficulty we choose. And the special way the machines are constructed creates a hybrid motion that's a bit like running and walking and climbing stairs and cross-country skiing all at once, but without excessive impact to joints, which means we're less prone to injury.

So why not learn how to use one? If you can't figure it out for yourself, just ask. I'm sure there's someone who'll be happy to help you. That's another part of Fit Tip #8. The staff at your workout place are an aspect of the facility. Use them. That's what they're there for.

A lot of facilities offer a complimentary training session when you sign up. If that's the case, what are you waiting for? Take them up on it! What a great thing! Use your complimentary session to speak with a qualified trainer with whom you can discuss your personal fitness goals. Ask him or her to recommend a few basic exercises you can start to work with right away. Take notes. Ask questions. Own this process. Start to make it your own.

By the way, these days, I don't just stick to the treadmill. *I make sure to vary my workouts and use as many aspects of my exercise facility as I can.* There are two good reasons for that. The first is that I want to condition my body to do lots of different things. This way I'm working toward well-rounded fitness. I'm also decreasing my chances of injury by not working the same group of muscles day in and day out.

But the second reason I vary my workouts is actually more mental than physical. I do it to keep from getting bored. Look, I love my gym membership, but when the weather feels accommodating I've been known to go for a run outside just to switch things up a bit, to get some sun and fresh air.

Here's the principle once again: *Try doing different things instead of locking yourself into the same old routine. That keeps your workout fresh and fun.* And fun is something that's very important whenever you try to get fit.

In fact, I think fun is *so* important, I've made it into a Fit Tip:

Fit Tip #9: If It Isn't Fun, You'll Fail

Thumbs up-to the Volkswagen company for what I'm about to write. That's right, I said Volkswagen, the ubiquitous German car company. Their Beetles and Jettas and snub-nosed vans have all played a very strong part in American culture over the past several decades. So what does Volkswagen have to do with getting fit? Hang on for a second, I'll tell you.

A few years back, Volkswagen launched an ingenious advertising campaign for their new line of Blue Motion cars—cars whose operations served to reduce the environmental impact so often generated by automobiles. The marketing staff at Volkswagen knew that a popular misconception existed among consumers that you had to sacrifice performance when you purchased a car that was engineered to be environmentally friendly. So the marketers chose to steer their campaign in a totally new direction. They made the case that driving these new Blue Motion cars was not only good for greening the environment, it was also a lot of *fun!*

Fun was the difference. Fun was the key. Fun, the marketers said, is important. Fun initiates new behaviors. For instance, when we find ourselves doing something fun, we want to keep on doing it, right? Hours go by like minutes. Days whip by like hours. We find ourselves getting up in the morning, ready to go to work. We talk to our friends about how we're having so much fun and invite them to get in the game, as well. Fun can motivate. Fun can change. Fun helps buoy our spirits.

Volkswagen set out to prove that having fun can serve as a catalyst to change people's behavior. Having fun, when properly structured, can help us choose the right thing to do—and not just for ourselves, but for society at large. They called this theory (oddly enough) the Fun Theory. But before they could use it, they had to prove it. So they tested it using a series of simple but ingenious experiments.

The first experiment involved a busy subway station in Odenplan, Sweden. In this station, commuters who had disembarked from their subway cars faced a choice as to how they would reach street level. Would they take the flight of stairs, or would they take an escalator that ran right next to the flight of stairs? Taking stairs can be good for you, as we've already discussed. But the researchers set up some cameras and studied the patterns of foot traffic for a while. Do you know what they discovered? That's right. A lot of people were taking the escalator, which led to this question: *How could the researchers change people's behavior and get them to take the stairs instead?*

Enter the Fun Theory. One night, while the subway station was closed, a team went in and doctored the steps of the staircase to look like a giant piano. There were long white keys and smaller black keys, just like you'd see on a keyboard. Then the team rigged up a series of pressure plates attached to a sound-effects machine so whenever someone put their foot on a step, the step would let out a different musical note, as if the person were walking across the keys to a giant piano. Did you ever see the movie *Big* with Tom Hanks? Remember that famous scene where he plays the piano by dancing on a life-size keyboard? That's basically the same effect.

The researchers set up their cameras again and stepped away from their masterpiece as the station opened for business the next morning. They took a lot of film footage of people discovering the keyboard stairs, and this footage tells the whole story. At first, you could see that people were skeptical. It was written all over their faces. *What's this?* they seemed to be thinking. *A keyboard? Who did this? Where are the usual stairs?* But then a curious phenomenon began to take place.

The first person stepped on the lowest stair and the stair went BONG! (which is my word for a low C note). Shocked, she stepped on the next highest stair. The next highest stair went BUNG! (a D note). Intrigued, she stepped on a black key next, just to make sure that those worked, too. Sure enough, the black key went BANG! (musicians know this note as D sharp, also called an E flat). After that, we were off to the races (or the stairs, but you get the point).

That first pedestrian got the idea. She started walking up and down the stairs. Smiling. Tapping her feet. She was making noises. Playing around. Killing time. By any measure, she seemed to be hitting those steps just for (wait for it, here comes the punch line and you knew it was coming, so don't be alarmed). . . *fun*.

And this continued throughout the day. Pedestrians came to the steps in wonder and got the idea pretty quick. Parents brought their kids to see it. Elderly people smiled and shuffled their way through a range of notes. Some people hopped up and down on one foot like a hopscotch musical blast. Friends enlisted other friends to help them tap out simple songs. *Happy Birthday. Frère Jacques. Here We Go Round the Mulberry Bush.*

The final result: 66 percent more people chose to use the stairs instead of the escalator! Had fun really changed the way people behave? You bet it had, and much more than that—it had changed them for the better, by which I mean it got them to sweat. Got them to exercise.

But then the researchers turned their attention to public trash cans. Anyone who's been to a major city in any part of the world knows that litter can be a problem. But what if it could somehow be fun to throw your garbage into a bin? Would people be more inclined to do it? Again, the researchers concocted a plan, one that would prove their theory. This time, they rigged a public trash can so it made funny sounds whenever something was thrown inside. The researchers filmed what transpired, and here again, the tape tells the tale.

Passersby were totally stunned the first time they tossed their trash in the bin. But then came smiles and lots of chatter. Strangers talking to strangers. Barriers being broken. Conversations started. Once the novelty was established, people started to throw their trash away with excitement, even exuberance! Researchers were somewhat stunned when they worked their tallies out at the end of the day. They found that, in one day alone, people had placed more than 158 pounds of trash in the doctored, sound-producing bin. On average, that more than doubled the amount of trash collected in similar-sized bins positioned throughout the park— bins that hadn't been rigged to make sounds. Bins that weren't much fun.

Had fun really changed the way people behaved? Yes, it most certainly had. But this time their behavior had a positive effect on the overall environment, too. People were inspired to pick up after themselves. The area around the doctored trash can was noticeably cleaner than ever before.

Finally, researchers worked their magic on a recycling bin. Again, they rigged the bin so that it made a series of funny sounds each time you tossed in an empty bottle. The "bottle bank" became a sort of "bottle arcade," complete with flashing lights and a digital score readout. And guess what: That day, nearly a hundred people used that recycling bin. During the same period, a nearby undoctored bottle bin was used . . . well, only twice.

The conclusion? Fun can change people's behavior, and clearly for the better. (For more information on the Fun Theory, as well as to see how Volkswagen applies this theory to their cars, I recommend that you visit www.thefuntheory.com.)

So what does this have to do with you and your quest to lose fat and get fit? Plenty, I say. And that's just the beginning. Listen very closely. . .

We've talked a lot about changing your lifestyle. Well, you can't change your lifestyle without changing your behavior, right? But most people never lose their weight and never get in shape because they simply don't want to change. They think of change as something bad, something that will hurt. That isn't really the case of course, but it's almost impossible to convince someone of that. Unless they see that change as fun. From that point on, it's all downhill.

So how can you make a fit lifestyle fun? Here's where your personal creativity comes in, but I'll give you a few techniques I've used just to get the ball rolling.

Let's say you're on a treadmill at the gym or going for a walk near your home. *Walking*, you might say. *Wow, that's boring.* Well . . . is it? It doesn't have to be, you know. The question you must ask yourself is, *How can I make walking fun?*

I mentioned that, when I first started out, I used to watch the news a lot on one of those little TV screens they mounted at my gym (I admit it, I'm a news junkie. Watching the news for me is fun). But of course you could watch any program you like. Or a movie. You could read a book or a magazine. You could read your local paper. Walking on a treadmill is great like that. It allows you to multi-task.

But what if you're not at a gym, you ask? Or you're at a gym where there's no TV? Why not buy an inexpensive set of headphones and listen to your favorite music? You could also listen to books on tape and get caught up on your reading. What would it be like if you listened to recordings of your favorite comedian telling jokes while you walked? Or language lessons, if that's your thing.

One of my friends has studied French for years on his morning walk. Now he can hold an entire conversation in French. He married a woman who speaks the language. He talks to other people in French. He's made a lot of French friends. I find that amazing! He learned a language while getting fit. Talk about a twofer! Seriously, an inexpensive set of headphones can be your key to fun-filled fitness, be it indoors or out. *Très bien!*

Or why not combine your walk with the spirit of exploration? Have you ever really gotten out and walked around your neighborhood? Do you know every building and every business? Every little nuance? If you live in a big city, the answer is almost certainly no. But don't be fooled. You could live in a small town for most of your life and still not know it so well. Walking can cure that problem fast. Pick a different direction each day. Start walking. Look around. Get curious. Ask questions about what you see. Wave to people now and then. Make eye contact and smile. Getting fit is about a whole lot more than changing your body, you know. It could also be about making new friends. And really, what could be wrong with that?

What are you still doing here? Have you gone for a walk yet today? Get moving!

Fit Tip #10: Prioritize Your Health!

Here's something I want to impress you with. Once I got back from Duke, I locked myself into my wellness routine. That meant seven days a week, I was up at six o'clock in the morning and out the door and into my car. The gym came first. That was my rule and I absolutely loved it.

In fact, I think it's fair to say that, once I returned from Durham, my time at the gym became a central organizing factor in my life. I planned my whole day around the gym because that's how important my health was to me. And by the way, please note the distinction. I didn't say "how important losing weight was to me." I said: "how important *my health* was to me." Believe me, there is a difference. Again, losing weight is a short-sighted goal. Done right, healthy living is permanent.

I have never gone to the gym *just* to lose weight. I go to the gym to get and stay healthy, which is vastly more important to me. Being healthy means that you get to enjoy your life. Your friends. Your job. New people. New adventures. Yes, a by-product of being healthy is that your weight comes off and stays off. But it also means there's a smile on your face. It means that you respect yourself enough to put your health first. I want you to stop and think about that. I want you to remember the distinction between dieting and lifestyle. One is much more powerful. That's the one we practice.

So when I got back from Duke, I prioritized my health. That's the simplest way to put it. And that means a lot more than making sure I got to the gym. It also factored into how I structured my day to eat healthy meals. For instance:

- *I never once skipped breakfast.* That's a really bad idea. You've heard that old saw about breakfast being the most important meal of the day? Well, it is. Studies have shown it, too. Consider what's going on from a common-sense approach.

    Suppose you've had a restful night's sleep. Let's call that seven to eight hours. You wake up. Your body needs energy but you ignore it, you don't eat a thing and push on straight toward lunch.

Your engines are running on fumes (so to speak). Ask yourself: What would happen if you drove your car without fuel now and then? You know the answer to that, of course. So why should your body be anything different?

But now take a look at the behavioral effects that can be caused by skipping breakfast. Suppose you don't eat a thing until lunch. By midmorning, you're probably ravenous. It probably takes a lot for you to focus on even the simplest tasks. Countless studies have shown that memory, cognition, even dexterity levels can suffer when you haven't eaten. So can good decision-making. And here's a danger that's much more subtle. *If you haven't taken the time to eat breakfast, by the time lunch rolls around, you're so hungry, you become less discriminating about what you eat.*

Someone offers a cream-filled donut? You say: *Sure! Well, why not?* Or: How about that candy bar? *Great. No problem. Give it here.* You'll do anything for energy. You'll put anything into your stomach.

But by eating foods that aren't wholesome, foods that have less nutritional value, you're plunging into a vicious circle of calorie-rich, non-fortifying meals that eventually tap you out. Going back to our engine analogy, that's the equivalent of running your machine on tar instead of on high-octane fuel.

By the way, the research on all this is clear. A study from Harvard Medical School conducted by Dr. Mark Pereira and several of his colleagues showed that people who eat breakfast each day are one-third less likely to become obese. One-third! As if that weren't convincing enough, the study also found that people who skip breakfast are twice as likely to develop problems with their blood sugar levels. Problems with blood sugar levels lead to increased risk of developing diabetes, as well as high cholesterol, a leading cause of heart disease. And this is just the beginning.

Let's cut to the chase. Do not skip breakfast! Plan your work, then work your plan. Keep your house stocked with simple foods that make for a healthy breakfast. Yogurt. Fruit. Bananas. Oatmeal. Eat these foods in the morning and your day will start just fine. Eat nothing, or eat unhealthy food? You'll reap what you have sown.

- *I almost always made my own lunch.* Yes, breakfast is the first most important meal of the day. But lunch can be just as important. A good healthy lunch is essential for boosting your mid-day energy levels when they're most likely to sag. A healthy lunch keeps your metabolism running strong until the evening.

Making your own lunch is a big part of Duke's training. Good old-fashioned brown bagging puts you in touch with the foods you eat. You control the portion size. You control the calorie count. You control the diversity. You become, as the staff at Duke so often stressed, the architect of your wellness. You stick to the plan.

I recently read about an interesting study that tested the brown bagging phenomenon. Nineteen women in Minnesota were asked to eat boxed lunches every day for two months, but they were given a choice between eating small lunches (767 calories a day) and large lunches (1,528 calories a day). Once they made their choices, they could eat as much as they wanted.

Guess what this study found out. The women who opted for larger lunches consumed about 278 more calories a day on average. These women also experienced weight gain. So what does that indicate? Simple, really. *Give a person the option to eat more and they will.*[22] By the way, this phenomenon is called *upselling.*

And guess who already figured out that people like to be *upsold?* You guessed it: fast food chains and movie theater concessions stands. Upselling is the notion behind super-sizing products. Popcorn. French fries. Soft drinks. Shakes. It's also a dangerous trap to avoid for consumers who want to stay fit. Making your lunch puts you in control. I still try to do it each day.

One last good word about brown bagging: Boy, does it save you money! You can wrap up last night's leftovers. Throw in a single-serving cup of healthy applesauce (I love those). Literally, there are hundreds of ways to stretch your dollar while making your lunch. When you do this, you're conserving your wealth while getting fit in the process. And really, what could be wrong with that?

Reintegrating My Life

Once I returned to my hometown from Duke, I started working with Chuck again. This time I wasn't behind the wheel of a Ford Econoline van—I was working at Chuck's office, which was at the statehouse in Trenton. And this was great because I finally had a solid eight-to-five job. No more twenty-two-hour days. No more driving all over the state. No more meals on the run. Don't get me wrong, the work was demanding. But at last, I was leading a structured life, and this was very important.

I would wake up every morning, get into my car, and drive myself to the Y. Every morning. That was the deal I made with myself. These days a lot of fitness experts will probably say that I should have taken one or two days off a week. And who knows? Maybe they're right. But I was driven. I'd set my goals. Besides, I was having lots of fun. I loved that I had time in the morning to catch up on the papers. I loved how *good* I felt in the morning after I'd walked for a while. So I did my workout, took a shower, got back in the car, and drove to work with my brown bag lunch riding shotgun.

As far as meals went, I pretty much ate the same thing every day. *WARNING: Given what I've told you so far, some of the things I ate will probably shock you.* We'll deal with that in a minute. For now, I want to stress one thing:

> *Meals are up to you. Once you know the basics of what foods are right for your lifestyle, you can tailor your menus however you like (I know I certainly did). Get creative! Personalize what you eat to your individual schedule and specific needs.*

I pretty much ate the same thing every day. For instance, breakfast was:

- 1 mini raisin bagel

- 1 banana

And lunch was usually this:

- 1 cup of instant noodle soup. You know the kind I'm talking about. Pour hot water into the cup. Tear open the chicken flavor packet, mix it in, and stir. *Voilà*. You have soup!

- 1 mini whole-wheat pita with mustard and a slice of low-fat lunch meat packed inside. Ham or turkey. Didn't matter. I alternated a lot.

- 1 cup of sugar-free applesauce. Like I said, I love little applesauce cups. You can buy them in any grocery store. They're nutritious and affordable, their foil seal keeps them fresh, and they always come in pre-measured portions. What could be better than that?

For dinner, I almost always ate:

- bagged salad with low-fat dressing

- a low-fat frozen meal

So let's pause here a moment, because a lot of you are probably a bit confused by now. You might be thinking, *Wait a minute. Aren't some of those items* processed *foods? More importantly, aren't they the* same *kinds of processed foods you told us to stay away from? Lunch meats, for instance. Frozen dinners? Baroni, what's going on?*

Well, yes. As a matter of fact, they are. Each of the foods I've mentioned above (with the exception of whole-wheat pitas and applesauce) is high in sodium. And yes, you've heard me go on and on about how detrimental high sodium levels can be to your physical fitness. How it leads to bloating and high blood pressure and plenty of other problems besides. So why did I eat these foods? Because they satisfied two out of three requirements that I wanted the food in my plan to have back then. Yes, they were all high in sodium, but:

1. they were *expedient* (meaning simple to make, not to mention fast), and

2. they gave me *a high degree of control over the portion sizes of meals*

The expediency part should be easy to understand. Those cups of soup took only a minute or two to prepare each day, and I liked that. A minute or two to pause and make soup fit perfectly with the busy pace of my workday at the office. Same thing for the sandwich. Each morning, when I made my lunch, I'd unwrap a slice, fold it into the pita, add mustard, and I was done. What could be simpler than that? And frozen dinners? Pop one into the microwave oven, press the buttons, wait two minutes, and *bing!* Dinner is served. For someone who isn't that great of a cook, these options allowed me to eat very well, and without a whole lot of effort.

Now let's talk about portion sizes. Eating these foods I've told you about made tracking my portion sizes easy. I never had to bother with weighing my food to make sure I was only having five ounces of lean red meat for dinner or six ounces of boneless, skinless breast of chicken, for instance. (In an ideal world, I'd have time to do that, but I'm sure you're already well aware that the world is not always an ideal place). Every single product I used had nutrition information clearly marked on the side of its package. That way, I could tell at a glance how many calories I was taking in, how much fat, and so on. I could tabulate things pretty quickly, and of course there was never any question that I'd end up eating more than I'd planned for any given meal. It was one slice of lunch meat.

One cup of soup. One frozen dinner. And so on. And I could easily keep everything counted in my food diary.

So yes, I could have eaten healthier those first few months after leaving Duke. But this is exactly what I mean about personalizing your lifestyle. I saw my relatively high-sodium diet as a compromise between convenience and strict adherence to what I'd been taught at the DFC. Sure, high sodium count is never really desirable, but I knew I was working out every day and drinking plenty of water. That's not an excuse, that's just what I planned. Your plan can be something different.

By the way, keep this in mind: This was back in the earlier part of 1995 before the bottled water craze. So I got my fluids the old-fashioned way. I went to the sink and filled up a glass from the tap and I drank it. Simple. I did that several times a day at the sink in my office kitchen. At home, I liked to drink Crystal Light. Still do, as a matter of fact. Another processed food? I guess. But not dangerously so. The DFC served Crystal Light. It was one of those beverages the staff at Duke listed as having negligible sodium and calorie counts. We were even told that recording servings of these beverages in our food journals was optional.

So what I'm saying is this: Are there better meal choices out there than the ones I implemented my first few months after Duke? Of course, and I urge you to do better than I did on this score! Use your creativity! Personalize your plan. If you've got the talent and time to cook, you can probably stick to a *much* healthier meal plan than I ever did. People who know how to cook healthy and who can build time to cook into their daily lives are usually way ahead in the fitness game. Frankly, I wish I was one of them.

Now people often ask me if I ever got hungry eating this way. The answer? Nope. Not really. I wouldn't say hungry. However, I *would* say that I looked forward to meals (the way healthy, fit people do). It's healthy to have an appetite. It shows that your body wants to be fed and wants to stay alive.

Calorie Counting: An Exercise

et's run through this exercise so you get a feel for exactly what I was doing. That way you can do it yourself, or something very similar to it. Remember, this is your plan, not mine. Tailor it however you wish. Once you get the basic idea, the rest is up to you.

Like I said, I jotted down everything I ate every day in my food journal. My food journal also served as my exercise log, but we'll get to that a bit later. So what was a typical entry like on a typical day in my journal? Well, let's take a look:

Breakfast

1 mini raisin bagel	120 calories
1 banana	About 105 calories

Lunch

1 cup of instant noodle soup	About 50 calories
1 mini whole-wheat pita	70 calories
with mustard	10 calories (2 teaspoons)
and a slice of low-fat lunch meat	This could vary based upon the type of lunch meat I ate. Generally about 60 calories.
1 cup of sugar-free applesauce	105 calories

Dinner

1 prepared salad bag	About 15 calories
2 tablespoons low-fat dressing	40 calories

1 frozen dinner	This could vary. My dinners usually fell between 300 and 450 calories, depending on what entree I selected.

And remember, throughout the day, I also drank lots of water and coffee and Crystal Light, all of which carry negligible calories. And of course, I never wrote down "this could vary" in my food diary. Like I said, one of my key enticements to eat these packaged foods in the first place was to help me do a quick and accurate calorie count. I checked the side of each box and jotted down the calories for the meal I was eating right then.

Still, you can see that I routinely ate about 1,200 calories per day in my basic meal plan. With a few snacks thrown in (a banana here, a packet of low-fat pretzels there), that amount rose to 1,500 or so. That amount, consumed consistently and coupled with a program of regular, moderate exercise, aimed me in the right direction to get me fit and keep me that way.

But then a very big hurdle popped up. I want to make sure you know about this right now so that you can avoid it, too. This really big hurdle I'm talking about was something I nowadays like to call:

Thank God It's Friday
(Now What Do I Do?)

Remember, I finally committed to losing my weight when I was twenty-two years old, a time when one's friends and social life are especially important. I love my friends dearly. We're very close. Over the years, we'd proven that we would support each other through anything. Still, I was nervous. How would my new goal of losing weight and getting fit affect the way that I used to cut loose? In essence, I was asking myself: *If I want to get fit, can I still go out with my friends? Can I do it the same way I used to do? Do I get to keep my social life while maintaining the goals that I've chosen?*

The answer is: You bet I could. But before I explain how, let me take a moment to tell you about the obstacle I faced in detail.

I don't know the kind of crowd you run with, but back when I was twenty-two, my friends and I would hit a string of bars and restaurants almost every Friday or Saturday night. A normal night on the town might involve getting pizza, burgers, chicken wings, and cheese fries, not to mention beer and possibly cocktails here and there. We abhorred the thought of driving while under the influence so one of us would always volunteer to serve as that evening's designated driver. The position used to rotate a lot but it never carried a stigma. In my group, fun came first; the alcohol was secondary. So even the designated driver ended up having a lot of fun.

When I got back from Duke, I did a series of quick calculations. I determined that each time I went out on a weekend night, I might end up ingesting between 3,000 and 4,000 calories. That's 3,000 to 4,000 calories *on top of* what I'd eaten for breakfast, lunch, and sometimes dinner.

And all of those calories were consumed late at night, shortly before I would go to sleep. That left my body very little or no time at all to stay active and digest the food. So it sat there like a lump in my stomach, making me slow and lethargic.

At Duke, I'd stuck to a regimen of 1,200 calories a day. And like I said, that figure had risen to about 1,500 once I'd arrived back home. Well, I was holding to that number—sticking with my plan. It was tough, but I was doing it. My new lifestyle was working for me. But I knew that, in order to keep that up, some changes would have to be made.

I had to find a way to have a healthy weight-losing lifestyle while still having an amazing group of friends. And that presented a challenge, of course, since my group of friends often went out to eat, though we weren't always on the same page with our lifestyle goals. So I found myself brainstorming about places we could all go to have a good time and relax. Surprisingly, I found several venues that offered lifestyle friendly fare.

One of the places we used to frequent was a Chili's on Route 1 near Princeton. The original draw for us were the beer and margarita specials, but I looked at the menu one night and noticed the section called the Guiltless Grill. *Huh*, I thought. *Perfect!*

Chili's could grill me a chicken breast with a side of steamed vegetables. They had a whole range of tasty salads (which I ordered with balsamic vinegar, no oil). Basically, they had food for me, for people who followed my lifestyle. I could work with what they were offering. They also had food that my friends could eat (which was basically everything else).

I started asking questions at all of my favorite haunts. I'd beckon the waiter over and ask, "Hey, can your kitchen do *this* for me?" or "What kind of meals do you have that are healthy?" And that's how I discovered the low-fat chicken sandwich at Chili's, or the pasta and grilled chicken plate at the local T.G.I. Fridays. In fact, that's when what I learned at Duke really began to kick in. The notion some people like to tout that you can never go out and eat healthy began to evaporate like mist. It's simply not true. You can have your whole new life (and eat it, too).

But the real challenge reared its head in the form of Italian food. I've always been wild for Italian food. My father makes a wicked lasagna. Plus, I grew up on the outskirts of Trenton, New Jersey. At one point, the Chambersberg section of Trenton had some of the best Italian restaurants in the country. Name a classic Italian dish and it's probably one of my favorites. For me, eating Italian food came as naturally as breathing.

But of course I needed to find a way to balance my new lifestyle with what I love to eat. What did people expect me to do? Boycott my favorite Italian places in order to make myself fit? Nope. No way. Denying yourself something never works. That's Diet Thinking, remember? Instead, let me show you how it works when you switch to Lifestyle Thinking.

The fact is, you can walk into any Italian restaurant in any part of the country and order something healthy. You can eat comfortably without sacrificing any of your goals. Remember Fit Tip #5? When Eating Out, Ask and You Will Receive. All you have to do is state exactly what you want. Look the waiter straight in the eye and say, "Hi there. How are you today? Here's what I'm in the mood for. A bowl of pasta and diced tomatoes, with a side of steamed broccoli, no butter. Can you do that for me? Thanks."

This became a running joke at Marsilio's, a place I used to go to a lot in Chambersberg. The staff started calling my usual order the Baroni Special. I'd walk through the door and the waiter knew exactly what I wanted. They understood what I was trying to do—they'd seen me going from fat to fit and were very supportive, which meant a lot. Support is what we're looking for.

When I first got back from Duke, I admit I'd sometimes stay away from restaurants whose menu I wasn't comfortable with. Now? It's very hard to find a restaurant I *won't* visit. Ninety percent of the time, I'll find something to eat that works for me. In fact, these days, my friends have a running joke. They say I'm very predictable and order the same entrees.

"Of course I do," is what I'll say. I usually don't explain more than that. If I did, I'd probably assure folks that I spend a lot more time thinking about food *after* having gone to Duke than I ever did *before*. I pay more attention to what goes into my body instead of just packing it in there.

I prefer low-fat, low-sodium proteins and almost always order fish. Fish is so dependable. It's low in calories but packed with protein, which is essential for healthy muscles and tissues. Fish contains plenty of essential minerals such as iron, zinc, and selenium. Fish varies in texture as well as in taste to give you lots of variety. Omega-3 oils, which are especially prevalent in fatty or oily types of fish, can reduce your overall cholesterol count, which protects your cardiovascular system while also reducing your risk of contracting certain cancers. Sardines, herrings, and mackerel are all really high in omega-3s. But you'll also derive great benefit from eating albacore tuna, lake trout, and salmon. Boy, do I love salmon! I could order it nearly every night and never get tired of it.

I also eat a lot of sushi. I just love the stuff. In fact, I often go out to sushi restaurants. The food is great and there's always plenty of other fare on the menu for people who don't like sushi. One of my favorite restaurants in New York City is 5 Napkin Burger in Hell's Kitchen. I think it's a perfect place. They have amazing burgers, but they also have a sushi chef on staff. So my friends can have a burger and fries and I can have my sushi. And the staff is so considerate there—they already know what I'm going to eat before I walk in the door.

Let me pause here and say this (it's important). By now, you can see that I like to eat healthy. *And my evening isn't any less fun because I'm eating healthy.* Eating healthy makes me feel good. Being with friends in a great atmosphere makes me feel good. That's what I get from going out to eat, the real charge, the spice, the life.

These days, I generally know what I want for dinner before I walk into a restaurant. How do I do it? Simple. I get proactive and use my tools. If the restaurant has a website, you can go online, check out the menu, and craft a few healthy options you can order when you arrive. That'll really put you at ease. Or who says you can't call ahead to discuss what they're serving that evening? Ask what vegetables are in season. Ask if their chef can cook your entree without any butter or oil. Check to see what substitutions can be made so you end up with healthy, delicious sides instead of something greasy or fried.

Remember: A restaurant *wants* you to be happy. They *want* you to have a great experience so you'll keep coming back again and again. So help them to help you out by taking charge of the situation. There's almost no restaurant that won't go the extra mile if you offer to walk it with them. Give them clear instructions. Eating out becomes a snap when you know what your body needs to be fit and ask the right kinds of questions.

So very soon after leaving Duke, I was out with my friends and enjoying life the same way I always did. Well, okay. That's not really true. I'm leaving out something important. Like I said, when I left Duke, I sat down and crunched some numbers. And this led me to make what I call a very important discovery. This very important discovery led me to make a big decision. And this becomes my very next Fit Tip, which is:

Fit Tip #11: Reduce or Eliminate Alcohol (or "Why I Quit Drinking")

I know, I know. I bet I just turned a lot of you off. No problem. I can live with that. But let me take a moment to explain myself before you close this book and walk away.

If you currently drink, I recommend that you reduce your alcohol intake in order to lose weight. I also recommend that you take a serious look at the role that alcohol plays in your life.

Believe me, I have my rationale for saying this. Basically, it's this: *If you want to lose weight, there's no better way to do it than to cut out or limit your alcohol intake.*

Did I used to drink? Yes. When I was in college, my friends and I would sometimes go out until two o'clock in the morning. We'd have a few drinks and after that, we'd stop someplace for a bite to eat. Sometimes we went to the local Roy Rogers. Sometimes we called to have pizza delivered. Sometimes we went to the Georgetown Café where we'd order eggs and pancakes and sausage and milkshakes and burgers and fries. Hardly a healthy lifestyle.

Yes, I'm aware that taking a drink once a day (or two if you're male) can benefit your HDL, otherwise known as high-density lipoproteins, the so-called "good cholesterol." I also know that if the alcohol you're drinking happens to be red wine, you'll ingest some powerful antioxidants. In fact, studies show that a glass of red wine can have hefty curative properties. These antioxidants I mentioned play a key role in combating cancer, aging, diabetes, heart disease, you name it. And some other very interesting studies point out that regular, limited alcohol intake can sharpen mental ability, especially in elderly patients whose mental acuity frequently wanes.[23]

But as compelling as all that certainly is, for me the risks outweighed the gains. Remember, I enrolled at the Duke DFC because I felt like my very life was in jeopardy. So what was more important for someone like me? Drinking a few glasses of alcohol to stave off the *possibility* of disease? Or losing weight, which would *almost certainly* make me healthier. For me, that was a no-brainer.

At Duke, I began to look at alcohol as just another mathematical component to my daily calorie intake. Some classes we took at the DFC helped to acquaint us with the calorie content of various alcoholic drinks. I've listed a few approximations for you below:

Drink	Approximate Calories
1 oz. shot of liquor (distilled, 80 proof)	65
Cocktail (e.g., Martini, Manhattan, Margarita)	160
12 oz. glass of regular beer	150
12 oz. glass of light beer	110
4 oz. glass of red wine	80
4 oz. glass of white wine	75

Duke taught us that, next to pure fat, alcohol has the highest calorie count per gram of anything you can ingest.* And of course, alcohol wasn't served at the DFC. It was never a menu item. During my first four-week stay in Durham, I discovered that *not drinking made it easier for me to hit my target intake of 1,200 calories a day.* And of course, as I've told you, a few weeks later, I actually started to lose weight.

Is it really such a drastic decision to stop drinking alcohol? Not when you're coming from my point of view. Once I started to lose my weight, I began to review the process that got me there. For instance, I thought, *Well, now that I've learned about how damaging fast food can be, I'm certainly not going to eat* that *again.* I'd determined that fast food had no role to play in my new healthy lifestyle, so I dropped it and never looked back. And the same went for alcohol.

If alcohol wasn't helping me lose any weight . . . if it wasn't helping me get fit and stay fit (and it wasn't) . . . I couldn't think of a reason to keep drinking it. So I didn't. It's as simple as that.

Now let me be clear about this. I don't want you to think I'm some crusader climbing up on his high horse and screaming that you should never enjoy a glass of wine with friends or drink a glass of champagne at a wedding. Absolutely not. Many people who want to lose weight and keep it off still take an occasional drink. *But I do insist that you drink responsibly.* I should explain what I mean by that, since it might not mean what you think.

Yes, I think that drinking responsibly means you should never get behind the wheel of an automobile after you've had a few beers. That's obvious. *But I also think drinking responsibly means that you understand how using alcohol impacts your overall health, as well as your goal to get fit. It means that you should understand what alcohol does to your body. And you should make intelligent choices about how it does or does not integrate with the rest of your new healthy lifestyle.*

Don't get me wrong, I still go out and enjoy myself. But I do it while sticking to my lifestyle goals. I do it without having to sleep late the next morning. No more hangovers or bloodshot eyes. I can go out late and

Bill's note: Proteins and carbohydrates contain about 4 calories per gram, alcohol contains about 7 calories per gram, and fat contains about 9 calories per gram.

have a great time and get up early the next morning and get to the gym before breakfast. I can get on the treadmill and read the papers or whatever book I'm into.

I'm often asked how my friends reacted when I stopped drinking. For the most part, very well! From their perspective, they now had a guaranteed designated driver!

But not everyone is going to understand the choices you make as you start to get fit. I think it's fair to say that some people I knew didn't understand why I stopped drinking, the same way some people didn't understand why I'd started getting up every morning and going to the gym at six. To them, that was very un-Bill-like behavior. But I didn't make those decisions for them. I made those decisions for me. And that brings me to my next Fit Tip, which is:

Fit Tip #12: Yes, It's Okay to Be Selfish Sometimes

Losing weight and getting into a healthy lifestyle is the single most selfish thing you can do. "Selfish" meaning "for the self." In other words, by getting fit, you're putting your*self,* your physical and mental well being, first on the list of importance. And as far as I'm concerned, that's exactly where it should be.

I understand how this might be confusing. When somebody calls you selfish, it's not a good thing about 99 percent of the time. In fact, these days, it's sort of become accepted to use the word *selfish* as a synonym for *self-indulgent.* One thesaurus I checked lists a bunch of other words that are similarly unflattering. Selfish can mean *egotistical, mean, narrow-minded,* and *narcissistic.* Again: That's not a good thing.

But you see *the 1 percent of the time when I think it's okay to be selfish is when it concerns your health. In fact, I submit that you should be selfish about your health.* Remember, I said *selfish,* not *indulgent.*

Let's review the difference a moment. Remember how I used to go out at midnight feasting on fast food in Hackettstown? That was indulgent. It was outright hedonism with food. No good was going to come from it.

Now compare that behavior with me saying that *I'm going to stop eating things that aren't healthy for me.* Or saying that *I'm going to take care of myself and exercise and put my health as one of my top priorities.*

You see what I mean? Now that's what I call being selfish, and you know what? I'll take it. I think it's a *good* form of selfishness and I urge you to consider it.

And I can share this with you: I've had people say to me, "Come on, Bill! Just have one drink. Will that make such a big difference?" Or: "Come on, Bill! One fast food burger. How could just one burger hurt? It's not like you're going to put 135 pounds back on in one afternoon, am I right?"

Of course they're right. But that isn't the point. *I have chosen not to do these things. And my choices are working for me.*

Remember what the diet industry wants us to think. It wants us to think that there's some magic bullet out there that will work for everyone and help us all to lose weight. But that doesn't make any sense. In fact, I'll repeat what I told you way back at the beginning of this book. I said:

> *Weight management isn't a cookie-cutter system. What works for one person might not work for another. The weight you carry results from a number of highly personal factors. So the way you lose the weight must be highly personal, too. You have to learn what works with your body, your mind, and your motivations.*

So . . .

Finding the way that we can lose weight . . . finding the way that we can stay fit . . . that's a very personal process. And I think it should be of prime importance because our very lives depend on it. If some people say that's a bad point of view to take, so be it. We can disagree.

All I know is that, once I realized I wanted a healthy lifestyle, nobody was going to dissuade me from going after it and making it mine. And I wish the same for you.

A Funny Thing Started to Happen . . .

I hope that nothing I've written so far makes you think that my weight just melted right off, like one moment I woke up and got out of bed and thought, *My! Look at that! My waistline is suddenly 32 inches!*

That would have been nice, but it didn't happen that way, not by a long shot.

I didn't expect it to, of course. The staff at Duke had taught me well. Specifically, they'd taught me that walking the road of success doesn't end. The end is never the goal. Walking the road and walking it well—that's the point, and nothing else.

So that's what I did. I walked the road—quite literally, as things turned out. Each day I got up at six o'clock in the morning and went to the YMCA and got on a treadmill and hit the start button and put one foot in front of the other. Day after day and week after week. Walking. Pretty simple, right?

In the beginning, I could only walk for twenty minutes. I looked up at the TV, which played CNN morning news. When the twenty minutes was over, I was winded, really spent. I jotted down what I'd done in the exercise journal I kept (and no, I haven't forgotten, don't worry, we'll get to that in a bit). And that was all. I was done for the day. Twenty minutes of exercise.

I would hit the showers and go to work. Get ready for the rest of my day. Days became weeks and weeks became months, which passed by pretty fast.

But then a funny thing started to happen. Recently, I took a look at my exercise journals from the early part of 1995. And I noticed that I started to add a little incline to the treadmill after the first few weeks. Not much. I punched in a factor of 1 on the treadmill's onboard computer. But then my journal tells me that I started staying on the treadmill for twenty-five minutes. And later I punched in a 2 on the treadmill's incline scale. And then I stayed on for thirty minutes. And so on.

A couple weeks later, I started to jog. Just a little, according to my journal. In fact, my notes indicate that I jogged for only five minutes the first time. But a few weeks later, I did it for ten. Then I added more incline. Then I added some more minutes walking. And after that, a few more minutes of running. And then a little more incline.

By April of 1995, my exercise journal says I was running through almost my whole workout. That's four months after I left the Duke Diet & Fitness Center. Me! The Fat Kid! I was *running*!

Now, this might be tough to articulate, but I have to try to say it. I remember that week at the DFC when I got on the scale and none of the weight had come off. I remember thinking I'd never lose a single pound, let alone the fourteen pounds I eventually dropped before I left Durham that first time around. That awful black hole of purest despair was one of the worst things I've felt in my life. So imagine my total astonishment when I finally lost some weight. I remember thinking, *I lost fourteen pounds! What next? Um, well . . . guess I'll try losing twenty!*

And that became my attitude. When I got to twenty I thought, *Okay, I wonder what thirty feels like.* And when I got to thirty I thought, *Okaaaaaay . . . what if I tried for forty?*

My journals tell all. On average, I lost one or two pounds a week. At that pace, very soon, my weight loss began to look pretty obvious. In fact, people started to comment about it. Better: They started to *compliment*!

I'd bump into old friends I hadn't seen in months or sometimes years, and someone would always make a remark like, "Bill! Man, look at *you*! You look really *great*!" Talk about inspiration! I'd get home from work at the end of the day and look at myself in the bathroom mirror and squint at myself, a little amazed. My face had begun to emerge bright and clear.

Part of me wanted to hop in the car and drive back up the turnpike. Back to that senior citizens' center I'd been to in Monmouth County. I wanted to find that woman who'd embarrassed me and show her what I had done. I also wanted to thank her, I guess. Because, in a very unusual way, she was my inspiration, too. *Remember: Not all inspirations are pleasant. Still, we can use them to grow.*

I didn't let up. I still went to the gym, every morning of every day. I stuck to my lifestyle. I stuck to my plan. Only now my plan was forced to include a lot of trips to clothing stores. I had to buy more pairs of pants, more shirts, and even a couple of suits. My clothes had started to hang like drapes. My shirts bagged out like sails without wind. The legs of my pants looked like unfilled sacks. I probably looked ridiculous, but I couldn't care less. I just smiled.

A word to the wise who wants to get fit: Yes, your clothes budget takes a big hit. So what? Odds are you won't mind in the least. The need to hitch your belt a bit tighter is proof that your lifestyle is working for you. And this is just the beginning. There is no greater feeling than seeing your clothes don't fit anymore.

Fitness Factors into Life Decisions

Since Chuck wasn't going to Washington (and I wasn't going with him), I started applying to law schools, and one of my top choices was Duke University. Duke Law School has a great reputation. And of course I thought how nice it would be to live very close to the center.

So the spring of '95 wore on and I started receiving acceptance letters from schools to which I'd applied. Nothing yet from Duke. But then I got accepted to the University of Virginia. I liked UVA and its reputation as an excellent school for law. Once I got my acceptance letter, I figured I'd drive down to Charlottesville and visit the school grounds during Admitted Students Weekend. Which turned out to be one of the best decisions of my life.

By that point, I'd dropped fifty pounds. You can bet that I was pretty excited to keep up my work and drop fifty more, which meant that I had to plan ahead. So during my trip to Charlottesville, I made sure to stay at a hotel that had a fitness center. And I made sure that this hotel stood next to a restaurant that I knew served healthy food. Although I was busy during the days—meeting people, touring the grounds, steeping myself in the atmosphere—I also made sure to get my workouts in. As it turned out, that wasn't very hard to do in Charlottesville, Virginia.

One of the things that I loved most about the town was how *active* everyone was! Everywhere I went, I saw people running, walking, playing Frisbee, tossing a football, getting out and having fun. And it wasn't just in one place—it was everywhere, all over the grounds. Immediately, I felt at home. I thought, *This is a place where people share the same set of values as me.* And this was very encouraging. Because in April 1995, although I'd lost fifty pounds, I wasn't where I wanted to be—not yet, at any rate. My lifestyle was certainly working, yes, but the road goes ever on.

And here's the kicker: The people I met in Charlottesville probably thought I was pretty big. But they had no idea how big I *used* to be, not the faintest clue. My body was changing, and with it, so was my attitude. I began to feel more optimistic. I started looking forward to things: my weekend, my school, my life, my career. I don't know how else to describe it. It was like a very big door had been opened and I was walking through it to meet the *me* I'd always imagined I could be. If that sounds sappy, so be it. It happens to be the truth.

I felt so satisfied with the lifestyle I found at UVA that I made my decision while driving home, all the way north to Hamilton, New Jersey. UVA had made me feel comfortable. So that's where I would go to law school.

I want to highlight something here: *I still felt like I was learning, still felt like there was room to improve.* That's a big part of Lifestyle Thinking, you know. The notion that *you're never finished, you're always in the game, always on the lookout for ways to live well, to feel better about yourself.* And one of my skills was put to the test that Fourth of July. It was my very first Independence Day after my very first visit to Duke. And yes, it presented a challenge to me, one that I hope you can learn from.

This skill I'm about to tell you about really helped me to branch out. It's basically the key to going anywhere at any time, to any kind of function, and being able to feel comfortable about your experience there. It's called:

Fit Tip #13: Bring What You Want to Eat to the Party

That very first Fourth of July after Duke, I was sharing an apartment with roommates and we wanted to have people over for a classic barbecue. You know the kind I'm talking about. Burgers and hot dogs out on the grill. Pounds and pounds of potato salad. A keg of beer on ice in a tub. Lots of laughter with really good friends.

I'd always loved a good Fourth of July—the summer, the history, the celebration. But how was I going to pull this off and stick to my goals at once?

The answer had nothing to do with fighting temptation or any of that. Again, that's a big part of Diet Thinking; I urge you not to go there. In fact, the more I thought things through, the more I had to smile. What was I getting so worried about? I was one of the hosts of this shindig! That meant I could plan the menu and offer the kinds of foods I liked, foods that are really healthy to eat. What could be simpler than that?

Yes, we ordered chicken wings, and yes, we ordered food for the grill. Hamburgers? Hot dogs? Check and check. Bags of potato chips? Corn chips? Beer? Check and check and check. But what about a nice green salad with dressing on the side? That way people could add what they liked. My roommates thought it over and nodded. Yes, that sounded good.

We also added chicken breasts. They're easy to cook and very healthy and delicious when you grill them. I also got us a nice fruit salad. Fresh fruit. Nothing canned.

Now you might be saying, *Bill, so what? You served what you wanted that Fourth of July because you were in charge of the party!* Well, if that's your attitude, I've got news for you. Ask yourself this: When are you *not* in charge of the party?

Suppose you're invited to someone's place and you don't know what kinds of food will be served. There's two ways to look at this situation:

- *The Dieter's Way*, which is: *Oh no! Good Lord, I'm trapped! I'm powerless to control my destiny! They'll probably have all types of food there that I'm trying to stay away from! Cookies and cakes and burgers and fries and stuff that will throw me off my game. I guess I'll just go and tough it out.*

Clearly, I'm having a bit of fun here. But some people find themselves thinking this way. I know, because I used to do it myself. But not anymore. It's counterproductive. I favor the second way of looking at this situation, which is:

- *The Lifestylist's Way*. It goes something like this: *My hosts certainly don't want me to feel uncomfortable. Therefore, I'll bring food that I like to eat and share it with everyone else!*

Why not be that thoughtful person who shows up bearing a vegetable platter? Yes, of course, you can even bring dip—for everyone else, not you. Or how about a selection of nuts that are plain, unroasted, unsalted? Nuts are an excellent, healthy snack. Or why not a fruit platter? Why not a salad? Munching on nuts and salad and vegetables helps fill your stomach with food that you like, the kinds that contribute to fitness.

WARNING: Do not be surprised if bringing this food to a party makes you a very popular guest. In other words, don't be surprised if you find that you're not alone in your goals to lead a healthy lifestyle. Other people are doing it, too. They'll like that you present them with choices conducive to optimum fitness.

The point is that you put yourself in control. Bring what you like to eat. Share it. Feel good. Help others feel good in the process.

But while we're on the subject of control, it strikes me that there's a lot more to say. For instance, here's another tip that I think you should really consider.

Fit Tip #14: Plan Your Snacks

I don't like to feel hungry. Frankly, I dare you to show me someone who does. And people get hungry throughout the day. It's one of those things you can bet will happen. *Unfortunately, it's also one of those things that makes a lot of people abandon common sense and eat whatever's available right then and there.*

And that often means that you're not eating healthy. And not eating healthy means not living fit. So I began to develop strategies to deal with my hunger pangs while still leading a fitness-oriented life.

I've already shared a few of these techniques with you. Drinking lots of water is one. Staying away from sweetened beverages and certain processed foods is another. But here's one that I find to be enormously effective: *Plan your snacks.*

For instance, people ask me all the time, Is it okay to snack when you're trying to get fit? Of course it is. Snacking is fine. You just have to do it sensibly. And that means keeping these four basic ideas in mind:

1. *Find things to snack on that are healthy.* We'll talk about some options in a moment.

2. *Make sure those healthy foods are available.* It's common sense that you can't lose weight while snacking on things like brownies and cupcakes. But common sense can go right out the window the moment we start to feel hungry. So don't let yourself get tempted. Keep healthy snacks with you at all times. Put them on your shopping list, buy them when you go to the grocery store, and keep some in your purse or your briefcase. Keep some at the office. Wherever you'll need them when you get hungry. That's the rule of thumb.

3. *Make sure that you count these snacks as part of your overall meal plan for the day.* Remember, a snack isn't a free pass. It's something you plan to nibble on to take away hunger cravings, but you still have to count it as part of your overall calorie intake for the day.

4. *Make sure that you jot down your snacks in your food journal.* Remember: Everything that you eat gets recorded.

So put this all into practice.

Suppose you're someone who always gets hungry in midafternoon. No problem. Find a healthy snack for yourself, make sure you've got it available, and budget that into your 1,500-calorie-per-day plan (if that's the goal that you've set for yourself—I'm using that as an example).

But wait. What kinds of foods make for healthy snacks?

Well, you can't go wrong with fruits and vegetables. Personally, I like little bags of baby carrots. You can buy them in almost any grocery store. Or celery sticks. Or grapes.

Or while we're at it, raisins! Raisins are great! They're packed with all sorts of vitamins and minerals like calcium, magnesium, phosphorous, and potassium. They're also a great source of fiber. You know those little boxes of raisins you used to eat as a kid in third grade? Each one carries approximately 125 calories. So they're easy to budget into your meal plan, delicious, and really filling. They're also convenient to carry around in a knapsack, a briefcase, a pocketbook, a coat. Keep those boxes of raisins around and you'll never go hungry again.

I'm also a *really* big fan of bananas. In fact, I eat them all the time. You pretty much can't go wrong with bananas. They're healthy, filling, and always available. They contain lots of vitamins C and B6, and all eight of the amino acids that are essential to good health, but that our bodies can't produce on their own. Bananas are also a great source of fiber, folic acid, and potassium. Did you know that two bananas can provide your body enough fuel for a tough ninety-minute workout? Did you know that bananas have been linked to alleviating symptoms of everything from depression, heartburn, and stress to ulcers, morning sickness, and anemia? According to the *New England Journal of Medicine*, eating bananas as part of your regular diet can reduce your chance of suffering a stroke by up to 40 percent. Plus, like all fruits, a banana comes in its own disposable, biodegradable wrapper. Now what could be better than that?

Sometimes I also snack on pretzels, a very healthy source of complex carbohydrates. They have lots of fiber and zero fat. You can buy them unsalted if you prefer, to lower your sodium intake. You can also buy them in those little snack pack bags, which controls the size of your portions.

And what's wrong with an apple? Apples have loads of fiber and they're a great source of vitamin C. They're low in calories (most apples are under 100) and also contain lots of vitamin B6, vitamin K, calcium, magnesium, iron—the list goes on and on. Studies performed by the National Cancer Institute show how eating foods such as apples (which contain a substance called flavonoids) can greatly reduce our chances of contracting certain forms of cancer. In fact, apples were cited as one of three flavonoid-rich foods (along with pears and red wine) that were shown to decrease mortality risk from causes related to cardiovascular disease and coronary heart disease.[24]

I could go on, but you get the idea. Let me repeat this important point: *Any fruit or vegetable that's easy to carry around with you or easy to get can make a good snack.* Thankfully fruits and vegetables are a pretty diverse subset of food. So get creative. Find what you like. Stock up on it and eat when you're hungry.

A word of caution: *Beware of snacks that claim to be healthy but really and truly are not.* Frankly, a lot of these products are manufactured to prey upon our quest for healthy food. And lots of people eat them as snacks thinking that this is a good thing to do when it probably isn't. In fact, I'm certain you can do better.

I'm very skeptical of protein bars, for instance. Health bars. Granola bars. You know the kind I'm talking about. A lot of them contain loads of sugar, and most are high in calories. Think of it like this: A chocolate marshmallow granola bar isn't your healthiest option. Yes, it has granola in it. That's nice. But the chocolate and marshmallow ruin the party. It doesn't make for a healthy snack.

The bottom line? Read the label first. Check your food journal. Check your plan. Then make decisions accordingly.

And here's some advice for people who travel. Don't wait to get out on the road to look for bananas and little pretzel packs. Don't assume you'll find healthy snacks at every roadside travel joint. Get proactive. Bring your snacks wherever you go. In the car. The airport. The bus. The train. This way, when you stop for lunch or dinner, you won't be so famished that you order something unhealthy off the menu. You can sit down and enjoy a nice salad instead. Or maybe an egg-white omelet (I could eat one any time of day—I really love them that much).

One other thing I'll say on this point: *There are times (I can almost guarantee this) when you'll find yourself somewhere, hungry, and without something to snack on.* Maybe your workout went really well that day and your stomach has started asking for more attention than you usually give it. Or maybe you're under a bit of stress and would like to have something to nibble on. Regardless of the reason, you find yourself hungry with nothing healthy to snack on.

That's fine. It really is. Remember, this is Lifestyle Thinking. You might have to make little adjustments here and there, but now that you know what to look for that's healthy, you can avoid the things that are bad for you and stick to what works best with your plan. If you absolutely must eat something that isn't particularly healthy, figure out what its contents are and jot the calories down in your food journal. Then try to learn from the situation. How can you have healthy snacks on hand if this ever happens again?

Food on the Run That Sticks to Your Plan

I already started to touch on this point in the previous section. Remember when I talked about bringing healthy snacks with you wherever you go? Especially for people who travel? Well, let's take a moment and put to bed a venerable (and incorrect) food myth.

Lots of people will say that you can never eat at a fast food restaurant and stay true to your fitness goals. That simply isn't true.

No, I'm not saying you can walk into McDonald's and wolf down a Big Mac. I also can't recommend Whoppers at Burger King, or about 85 percent of the food being served in chains like that. It's true: they're just not good for you. Even the so-called "healthy options" often listed on fast-food menus can run pretty high in fat, sugar, sodium, and calories.

But remember what we talked about when I described the Restaurant Experience. You've cultivated skills that allow you to weed out the dross that you'll find on the menu of nearly any establishment. Put those skills to work right away. Even in a fast-food place, you can look to order healthy.

And sometimes, I admit: you'll find yourself in a situation where you don't have much choice as to what you can eat. For instance, I remember one time I was working in Michigan in 1996. My colleagues and I found ourselves in a small town where the only place we could eat was the local Wendy's. I mean that literally, by the way. This town had only one place to eat. The Wendy's. That was it.

At first, I was concerned. I thought I'd have to adjust my eating habits. But then I took a deep breath and read the menu closely. *Well, well,* I thought. *Okay. No problem.* I ordered the baked potato, no butter, no sour cream, as well as the low-fat chili they served, which turned out to be surprisingly good.

Look, this could happen. You should bet that it will. Someday you might find yourself traveling. It doesn't matter what for. You might be moving around on business. Maybe you're off to visit old friends or take a family vacation. Lunch or dinner pops up but you're on the highway with limited options. Looks like the only solution you have is to visit a fast-food chain, or maybe some kind of diner. But DO NOT PANIC! These places have plenty of options for people like you and me. I've listed some of my favorites below.

Subway

We all know of the Subway commitment to healthy eating. Subway is one of the largest fast-food chains in the world. Primarily, they offer sandwiches, but most locations also offer salads and such. What do I love about Subway the most? They've taken the lead in their industry by disclosing the calorie content of nearly every item they offer. Their food is reasonably priced. And their ordering system allows you to craft a sandwich to your specific design.

I like the six-inch sandwiches. You can ask for all different kinds of bread, but I typically stick with their whole-wheat roll, which is fresh and very tasty. Here are some sandwiches I have ordered, along with approximate calorie counts:

Sandwich	Calories
Six inch turkey breast on wheat	280
Six inch deli ham on wheat	290
Six inch deli roast beef on wheat	320
Six inch veggie delight on wheat	230
Six inch turkey breast and ham on wheat	280
Six inch oven roasted chicken	320

With calorie counts as low as these, you can easily splurge and add a slice of cheese to your sandwich if you like (I don't, but the math says you can). Plus, another great thing about Subway is the way they let you load on the salad. What else would you like on your sandwich today? Lettuce? Onion? Tomatoes? Olives? Pickles? Cucumber? Spinach? How about green peppers? How about hot peppers? Banana peppers? Go ahead. Throw it all on. Don't stop. Subway always serves fresh vegetables, and all of them are good for you. Another quick suggestion? Stay away from the signature sauces and condiments like mayonnaise. Even the low-fat, low-calorie options can really throw you off your calorie counting game. Instead, I recommend mustard, which has no fat and packs in a lot of flavor, perfect on just about everything.

If I ever find myself out on the road, I always look for a Subway first, and always order healthy.

Wendy's

No, I don't order their Old Fashioned Hamburgers. Nor do I order their chicken sandwiches, nuggets, wraps, wings, or fish fillets. None of them measure up to my goals, but I have to say, there's nothing like a Wendy's baked potato when you find yourself on the road.

I always say no to the sour cream and chives topping. Likewise for the broccoli, bacon, and cheese options. Why? Because I know what's in a potato and I'm comfortable with that. Potatoes are a rich source of potassium, iron, phosphorous, and magnesium. Your average baked potato provides a delicious, filling 160 calories, give or take. But I don't always know how the toppings are prepared, and anyway, they're not essential to me. So just the potato, thanks.

Combine your baked potato with a Wendy's small serving of chili (another 225 calories or so) and you've got an excellent dinner or lunch. Wendy's also offers great salads you can order by the half size. Their apple pecan chicken salad is great, and only 245 calories.

Diners

I'm a Jersey kid, I *love* diners! *Love* them! Why, you may ask? Because most of them hand you a menu that's nearly as thick as Roget's Thesaurus. You can flip through the various pages and sections and cobble together a perfect meal, one that fits your needs completely and never leaves you hungry.

Diners serve breakfast twenty-four hours a day. That means you can always order an egg-white omelet, which is one of my favorite meals. Egg whites have no fat, no cholesterol, and practically no calories, but they serve as an excellent source of protein. What could be better than that? Add some chopped fresh vegetables like tomatoes, mushrooms, onions, peppers. Ask the chef to make the eggs in a pan without butter or oil. Now you've got plenty of vitamins, too, in a tasty, filling meal for under 200 calories.

I love the fact that I can walk into the Golden Dawn Diner in my hometown of Hamilton, New Jersey, at two in the morning or two in the afternoon and know that they're ready to give me great service, as well as a healthy meal.

Do diners have skim milk? Sure they do. Coffee? Of course, it's their stock in trade. They also serve plenty of fresh green salads—just ask for the dressing on the side. Diners also abound with vegetables. Green beans, baked potatoes, corn, peas—order whatever's on special that day. You can bet that a diner will also have plenty of boneless, skinless breast of chicken. Some of the bigger ones even have fish. Just ask to have everything cooked without butter or oil. Say no to bread. Have a glass of water instead of a cola. And always control your portion sizes.

By now, you probably see what I'm getting at. Even when you're on the road, you don't have to try to subsist on fast food. Don't order a pizza. Look around and get creative. Consider this situation a challenge. Commit more than ever to lifestyle choices. Your lifestyle, in turn, will commit to you.

Are you staying in a hotel? Fine. Don't give in and order room service. Apart from all the money you'll save, you won't find yourself at the mercy of cooks who might disregard your preferences.

If you're staying in the same place a few days, ask your hotel to put a little refrigerator in your room. Go to the front desk and ask for directions to the local supermarket. *Go out and buy your own groceries.* Try having cold cereal in the morning with skim milk, orange juice, and sliced fruit on top. Follow that up with a brown bag lunch—a sandwich that you prepared yourself, and maybe an apple or some kind of side like a cup of soup or some carrot sticks and hummus.

Make sure to buy plenty of snacks for yourself. Pretzel packs. Vegetable slices. Plenty of fruit. If your hotel has a microwave you can use, I recommend buying mini-packs of microwaveable popcorn. Popcorn is filling, a great source of fiber, and tastes really great. Plus one of those little mini-packs has just over 100 calories.

Remember who's in charge when you travel. You are. This is your vacation. Your business trip. Your journey to visit friends. Whatever. Stick to your lifestyle. Get in the habit. The habit, in turn, will get into you.

Law School

started law school at the University of Virginia in August of 1995. Throwing yourself into anything new, especially a fresh course of study, typically demands energy. But that didn't feel like a problem for me. I found that I had energy to spare.

I loved my life in Charlottesville and I loved my classes at UVA. At the same time, I found out that I love the law, the logic of it, the reasoning, as well as the quest for justice in a world where justice so often is lacking. That kept me going day after day. Still does, as a matter of fact.

But something else was motivating me. *I was changing, re-creating myself. The process I had begun at Duke hadn't stopped. If anything, it had intensified!* Between April when I'd toured UVA and my very first day of class in August, I'd lost another fifty pounds (and change, but hey, who's counting?). Day by day, I kept losing weight. Week by week and month by month. How did I do it? That's actually simple: I stuck to the changes I'd made.

Exercise became a priority. It was as important to me as reading my law school books and writing my papers and meeting new friends. I built my gym time into my schedule. Often, I'd go to class in the morning, work out at midday, then grab lunch and take another class in the afternoon. I also varied things up a lot. For instance, I played on a softball team and also liked to go golfing with my closest friends. Active! That was the key for me! I found that I was enjoying my life in direct correlation to how active I was, a very important formula.

And how was I eating? That's actually funny. Because I remember thinking how tough it had been to eat healthy foods while gallivanting all over New Jersey on the campaign trail. Believe me, that didn't hold a candle to law school, and yet I continued to eat healthy meals! I made

164

healthy eating another priority. It wasn't hard to do. To me, it all boils down to routine, a very powerful concept.

Think about it. Our routines help to shape and define our lives. Healthy routines lead to healthy lives. Unhealthy routines lead to unhealthy lives. I had experienced both of these. For instance, my routine while I was driving for the Senate campaign was to get up every morning, drive to the coffee shop, and have donuts. Healthy? Nope. Not at all. A new routine was needed.

At UVA, nearly every morning, I got up and went to have coffee with a very special group at a cafe in the law school building. Bill Hagedorn, Bill Charron, Ann Ayers, Mary Lou Brown. We called these meetings Coffee Talk and we never had an agenda; it was totally informal. We'd sit and chat about politics, our studies, or current events. Whatever came to mind.

Often, I ate my breakfast then. A banana with some oatmeal, maybe. Or a bowl of sliced fresh fruit, or an egg-white omelet. Good friends, good food, good coffee, good talk. See, *that's* a healthy routine.

And I came to see that, in many ways, my selection of UVA law school was one of the smartest choices I'd ever made. Because UVA is sort of an antithesis to your stereotypical law school. Many great schools promote an atmosphere of intensity where students don't or can't make time for anything else but their work. But UVA has a different take. Yes, they have amazing professors at UVA, and yes, it's one of the greatest law schools in the world. But UVA follows the teachings of its founder, Thomas Jefferson. And Mr. Jefferson believed in ideals that are still pretty cutting edge to this day.

For instance, he very much respected the well-rounded individual. Someone, that is, who is healthy intellectually, healthy physically, healthy academically, and healthy socially. One cannot be forsaken lest the other attributes suffer. Balance always. That's the key. At UVA, that translates to quality of life that few schools (let alone law schools) can ever hope to touch. Of course academic work is important. But so is recreation. So is spending time at social events. So are your beliefs.

While I was a student at UVA, the university completed a new Aquatic & Fitness Center. And they posted one of Jefferson's quotes on the wall across from the front desk as you walk into the building.

> *Give about two hours every day for exercise, for health must not be sacrificed to learning. A strong body makes the mind strong.*
> —*Thomas Jefferson, 1785*

I took this quote to heart while I was a student. I take it to heart today.

Like I said, by the time I showed up to start classes at UVA, I had lost more than a hundred pounds. Sure, this felt great, but maybe the best part was that nobody at UVA knew me as Heavy Bill. Actually, I take that back. There was one person I'd gone to college with who also chose UVA law school. But that makes one person out of a total university population of approximately 24,000. In other words, it was a brand new world for me, and one that I found I enjoyed.

I had to get a whole new wardrobe before showing up at law school. New jeans, new pants, new shorts, new shirts. I'd started out as a 54 Long jacket with a 48-inch waist, and none of my clothes would fit anymore, no matter how much I took them in. By the way, let me tell you: *It's one of the greatest feelings in the world when you're getting into shape and your clothes don't fit anymore.* Not because they're too small. No, for the first time in my entire life, everything I wore was too big!

What a great feeling that is! There's no more tangible proof that your lifestyle really works.

By the end of my first semester at UVA, I was down to 185 pounds and change. That meant I'd lost over 130 pounds total, but better than that: I was keeping it off. I was down to a 42 Long jacket with a 33-inch waist. I'll say that again since it still makes me happy: I was a 33-inch waist!

Can you see yourself doing that? Sure you can. If I could do it, so can you. There's no great secret to getting fit and staying that way for life.

You just have to follow a few simple rules. This next one is one of my favorites.

Fit Tip #15: Set Goals (Keep an Exercise Journal)

If you don't know what you want, you'll never get it—that's a rule in life. But don't worry. You already know what you want. You want to drop fat. You want to get fit. That's your goal and it's very clear. So congratulations! Now that you have a goal, you can move to the second phase of the process: plotting how you'll *reach* your goal. But don't worry, that part's easy, too.

Here's a misconception I find that a lot of people have: They think that setting a goal has to be some awesome, groundbreaking, manifesto-style event, one where you totally rewrite the software of who you are and how you live your life. Does that sound dramatic? It does to me. Frankly, I find it a bit overwrought. In fact, if this is the way you normally think, I'd be a little surprised if you *didn't* have difficulty accomplishing things. You know why? You're setting your expectations too high. Biting off more than you can chew.

Slow things down a bit. Simplify. Remember that:

Setting and achieving goals is best done one tiny step at a time.

For instance, I know that you want to lose the weight and I know you'd like to lose it right now, but that simply isn't possible. But don't worry. The weight will start to come off, and pretty fast to boot. Just set yourself a few small goals. I bet you already have some. For instance, by now you probably see that some very effective small goals include:

- "Every day, I will write down everything I eat in my food journal."

- "I will learn to get to know my food by keeping track of calories."

- "I will set a daily calorie goal for myself and meet it consistently."

Goals like this are simple to implement. Simple to satisfy. They take care of one part of getting fit: controlling what you eat.

But now it's time that we set new goals for the other side of the coin. And that means *creating exercise goals*. And again, it's simple to do.

Just as before, we will not rush. We'll give ourselves an exercise goal that's small. Simple to obtain. That could be something like, "Right now I walk for twenty minutes whenever I get on the treadmill. But I want to walk for thirty minutes." Great. You've just defined your goal. Another small goal could be, "I'd like to go from exercising three days at the gym to five days at the gym." Fantastic. You've just defined for yourself the direction you want to go. You've set the goal. Now go after it. That's really all there is to it.

Regardless of what your small goals are, make sure to keep them obtainable.

Don't go too fast. Don't take too much. But *do* work slow and *do* have fun. That's how you stick to your plan.

Remember that twenty minutes on the treadmill *will* become thirty minutes. And fifty sit-ups *will* become one hundred. And one mile *will* become two miles . . . so long as you keep your goals small and obtainable. Then you work them one day at a time.

But now you might be saying, "Okay, I got the whole small goals thing. But what about my *big* goals?"

Well, look. Eventually, small goals build up to bigger goals. Which in turn build up to bigger goals. It's a question of degrees, and it only becomes a problem when we set big goals and insist that we get to them *now*.

For instance, can you imagine somebody saying, "Today my goal is to run a marathon," without having put any forethought and preparation into it? Nobody's done that since the first marathon was run by a Greek messenger named Pheidippides. He watched his army defeat the Persians, then he ran 26 miles and 385 yards and burst into the Athenian senate and proudly gasped, "We have won!" And then he died.

Yes, it makes for an interesting legend. However, it's hardly behavior to copy when trying to make yourself fit.

By the same token, no sane person would say, "This week, I'm going to lose twenty pounds." There's simply no way to do that. It's completely unrealistic. That goal is way too big for the allotted time limit. But remember: That doesn't mean we can't attain that twenty-pound goal over time. We simply have to set reasonable goals. Small goals. Then we obtain them. And then? We set new ones. We keep moving forward.

> *Plan your work and work your plan. That's how small*
> *goals build into big ones . . . big goals build into bigger*
> *goals . . . and on and on and on. That's the long-term*
> *chain of events, and that's how you reach success.*

So now we'll set goals for our exercise. It's simple. I want you to start doing this:

> *Start using your food journal as an exercise journal as*
> *well. Simply put, I want you to jot down the exercises you*
> *do each day to help you set goals for yourself.*

Let's suppose you've been taking a twenty-minute walk each day and then doing ten sit-ups. When you're finished, you'll jot that down in your food diary, next to what you've eaten that day. "Twenty-minute walk, Ten sit-ups." Now set a goal for yourself. Maybe you want to walk for twenty-five minutes by the end of two weeks. And maybe by the end of that period you want to be doing twenty sit-ups. Great. That's all you have to do. Keep that in mind and you're on your way.

Goals should always push you toward a higher level of lifestyle. That's my way of saying that you should always find yourself moving in the right direction. Keep the trend moving forward.

But look. If you find yourself hitting a plateau or especially challenged at any phase, don't worry. These things happen. And you're in luck. If you find yourself hitting a difficult spot, if you find yourself falling away from your lifestyle for any reason at all, you've already crafted a tool that will help to get you back on track.

Go back through your food journal. Find a period in the past when you were enjoying consistent progress toward your goals. Take note of what you were eating then, and what kinds of exercise you were doing, and in what quantity. Use that as your new starting point. It's like hitting the reset button. Start from there and move forward again as if the block never happened.

Working like this—from small goal to small goal—delivers consistent success. Eventually, you'll find yourself doing something you've planned to all along. And that's one of the greatest feelings in the world. It's that moment when you've just walked for forty-five minutes and you stop and say to yourself, "You know? I've never done that before!" That moment when you look back over your exercise journal after a few months and say, "Wow, look at how far I've come!" Moments like that open up all kinds of possibilities for us. They make us want to go even farther.

And one last thing before I forget: As much as you might be tempted to think it's about the goal, it's not. Keep in mind, that's Diet Thinking. The end is never the means. The really important part is the journey—what you do and how you do it and who you become as you seek your goal. Enjoy the trip. That's Lifestyle Thinking. The core of healthy living.

A Moment When Everything
Changed Again

In the spring of 1996, I'd reached the end of my first year of law school at UVA. I'd stuck to the lifestyle I'd started at Duke, honing it every now and then to accommodate new developments. Having surpassed a lot of old goals, I felt it was time to set a few new ones. So I told myself I'd enter to run the Charlottesville ten-mile road race.

I'd never done a road race before and I'd certainly never run ten miles. Sure, I was running a lot by that point, but three miles was my usual distance. In fact, I'd mapped a particular route I liked to take when I ran, one that wound its way from the UVA gym, through the grounds, then back to the gym again. That was my normal routine, but again, it was only a three-mile loop, nowhere close to a ten-mile course. Ten seemed totally out of the question, but that wasn't really the point.

I told myself that my goal was to finish—not *run* the whole course, just *finish*. I didn't care how I crossed the finish line. I figured I'd run until I got tired, then walk the rest of the way. That would be totally fine by me. Finishing was my goal.

So I went ahead and signed up for the run and checked in on the day of the event and got my number and pinned it to my T-shirt. The starting line was starting to get crowded so I headed over and found a spot and started to stretch out a bit, getting ready, limbering up. I had my trusty headphones on, and I was listening to a cassette tape of Beethoven. That's right, I said *cassette tape*. Remember those? I know what you're thinking. *My, how quaint!* Don't laugh. They used to be popular.

Pretty soon the officials called for everyone to get ready. The starter's gun went off with a *CRACK!* and everyone started to move. What an exhilarating feeling to be part of a pack of runners! That starter's pistol—and Beethoven's 5th —started a journey that was a metaphor for my weight loss.

I remember feeling strong for the first mile, the second, and then the third. *Huh*, I thought. *Okay. Pretty good.* My feet kept moving, kept covering ground, but this was nothing new. I'd run three miles before. But then the fourth mile spread out before me and I remember thinking, *Okay, this is something new. I'll probably start to walk any time. At some point, I'll get tired*, I thought. *At some point, I'll know when to quit. I'll stop and walk from there on out.*

But I didn't get tired. I kept right on running. And no one was more surprised than me.

The tape I had in my Walkman that day was one of those ninety-minutes jobs that used to switch automatically when it got to the end of a side. The mix I'd recorded started with Beethoven's 5th symphony and finished with his 9th. If you've never exercised to music, I wholeheartedly recommend it. Moving to your favorite songs can really help you enjoy yourself. Help you to have a lot of fun. Help you to stay really focused.

At one point, I looked up from the road and realized I was about to pass the ninth mile mark. And I remember thinking, *How can that be? Is this right? Why am I still going?* But I didn't spend a whole lot of time trying to figure it out because, by that point, I was starting to think, *You know what? I just might be able to finish this . . . I might be able to run all ten miles!*

Crowds had formed on the sides of the road to cheer the runners on. At that point, the race wound past the Rotunda where the UVA band had stationed itself. As I ran past, the bandleader pumped his arms and *BOOM!* The band kicked into a song.

I can do this, I thought. *I can DO this!* And I started to run the last mile.

The final stretch was full of hills, but I didn't care by then. I didn't strain or grunt or hurt myself to keep going. I think you probably already get my stance on hurting yourself. I just kept running. It felt really good.

My legs kept moving, and I got carried along. Up the hill, then down another. Up another, then winding down. I saw the finish line in the distance and went toward it.

People were cheering and screaming. Mind you, they weren't cheering and screaming *just for me*, but so what? It felt awesome, like getting a really cool gift. I accepted it—no, that isn't quite right. I *fed* off it. That's more like it. By that point, I could see the end of the goal I'd set out to finish. And after eighteen months of change—of hard work, dedication, and dreams—I don't mind saying how much I felt like I'd earned this victory.

Crossing that finish line was easily one of the best damn feelings I've ever had in my life.

Somebody asked me recently what my time was for that first ten-mile race. I don't remember the precise numbers, though I recall it was under ninety minutes. So, okay, I guess I'll have to admit: I'm no Jesse Owens. I'm Bill Baroni. But that race, for me, was the gold medal in my Life Olympics. I'd finished the course like I'd set out to do.

Not bad for a fat kid, I thought.

When it was all over, I wrote a letter to Dr. Hamilton and thanked him. Later the DFC ran that letter on the cover of *DFC Digest*.

But now that we're talking of exercise, it's time that you and I got more specific. So far I've kept my advice pretty simple, and focused on aerobic fitness. Aerobic means "with oxygen." Aerobic exercises are sometimes called cardiovascular exercise. We perform them for sustained periods of time to elevate our heart rates. Jogging for distances counts as aerobic. So does swimming and hiking and walking up stairs or down the street. The longer we keep our heart rates up, the more calories we burn, and the fitter we typically are.

But it's time to take our fitness goals to another, deeper level. It's time to add in anaerobic exercises. Anaerobic means "without oxygen." But don't get hung up on terminology. As far as you and I are concerned, anaerobic means *strength training*. And this becomes very important because the next Fit Tip on our list is this:

DFC Digest

http://dmi-www.mc.duke.edu/dfc/home.html

DFC Digest is the quarterly newsletter of the Duke University Diet and Fitness Center.

Please contact Brian Mack at the DFC, 800-362-8446, ext. 247 or mack0002@mc.duke.edu with news suggestions, questions or comments.

SUMMER 1996 • Volume 9 • Issue 2

Running for His Life!

DFC grad Bill Baroni reaches personal goals on the road to better health

A month at the Duke Diet and Fitness Center in November 1994 helped Bill Baroni put himself on the road to better health, literally. As part of his fitness program, this University of Virginia law student took up running, and recently completed a ten mile race! Congratulations to Bill, who shares his excitement in this letter to DFC Director Michael Hamilton, M.D.:

Bill Baroni

Bill stopped running long enough to snap this picture!

April 14, 1996

Dr. Michael Hamilton
Duke Diet and Fitness Center
804 West Trinity Avenue
Durham, North Carolina   27701

Dear Dr. Hamilton:

Greetings from Law School! Things are well here in Charlottesville, but I am looking forward to spending the summer back in New Jersey at home.

Classes are going well, but exams are approaching, and the studying is cutting in on my golf time! The good weather has allowed me to take my exercising out of the fitness center to the roads (and far too many hills!) of Charlottesville!

Speaking of that, I did something I never imagined I could do before I went to the DFC: run a ten mile race! It is hard for me to believe that less than two years ago I did not want to walk up a set of stairs, and yesterday I started the race just hoping to finish the ten miles -- and ended with me just barely running it under 90 minutes! Looking back two years, I can't believe I ever did not want to do this. Although I did not win the race (not even close) I did meet a new personal goal. Setting and reaching goals is what the DFC taught me, whether finishing the race, or keeping a healthy DFC-lifestyle. I have enclosed a copy of part of the official race results showing my not-so-near-the-top finish!

How are things going for you? Let me know how things are. I look forward to hearing from you soon!

All my best,

Bill Baroni
Bill Baroni

Bill Before

Fit Tip #16: Shed Pounds by Lifting Weights

I know this might sound counterintuitive, but the more weight you put on, the more weight you can lose. *Provided that the weight you put on is good, lean muscle weight.* This will probably take some explaining. It doesn't make sense to most folks who hear it for the first time. Until, that is, you understand a very important fact about the human body.

Muscles have the power to burn calories even after you've stopped exercising. Fat deposits do not.

Therefore, the more muscle tissue you have, the easier it is to burn off fat, even when you're resting. Let me explain how.

Remember what I told you before? The DFC taught me (and I'm teaching you) that losing weight is a simple equation—calories in versus calories out. At the end of the day, our bodies will store any excess calories (calories we haven't burned) as fat. By the same token, if we've burned through all of the calories we ingested and still need more, we're running a calorie deficit. Our bodies burn fat to make up the difference. That's pretty simple, right?

We also learned about keeping track of our calories. By now you should be logging your meals, writing them down in your diary, and making quick notes about how many calories they represent. Then, beside your meals each day, you should be jotting down the exercise you've done.

By the way, people often ask me: *How can I calculate the calories that I burn?* I guess they want to do a strict comparison of calories in versus calories out. But calculating the calories you burn during exercise can be tricky. In fact, it's such an inexact science that I've never really bothered with it myself. I'll try to explain why it's so imprecise, as well as why you don't really have to worry about it.

The basic problem has to do with something called metabolism. You've probably heard this word before. As far as you and I are concerned, metabolism refers to the biochemical process by which our bodies convert calories into energy. And the simple truths about metabolism boil down to this:

- Some people have a **high metabolism**, which means they burn off calories fast, and often with seemingly little effort.

- Some people have a **low metabolism**; this means their bodies burn calories slowly.

I'm sure you've overheard conversations where people celebrate or bemoan their metabolisms. That guy over there who looks fit and slim says, "I can eat whatever I want, my body burns it right off!" Meanwhile, everyone else in the room (the people like me) might be groaning and rolling their eyes. We might say, "It's not our fault that we gain so much weight—our metabolisms are low!"

It's true that everyone's body burns calories at different rates. It's also true that our bodies burn calories constantly, even when we're asleep. Think of all the reasons why. We continue to breathe when we're sleeping, don't we? Well, breathing takes a certain amount of energy. Our blood continues to circulate, right? Of course, and that takes energy, too. Our hearts keep pumping. Our brains keep dreaming. Our glands keep working to regulate hormones. And each of these vital processes requires a certain amount of fuel. In other words, our bodies must burn calories to power even the most basic functions of life.

The amount of calories we burn simply by being alive is called our Basal Metabolic Rate (sometimes abbreviated as BMR). Everyone's BMR is different—like I said, some have high BMRs and some people have really low BMRs. But whether they're high or low depends on three very important factors:

- *Gender*. Sorry, ladies. Men typically burn more calories at rest than women do. Why? Because men typically have higher muscle-to-fat ratios than women do. And since muscles can burn calories even when they're resting, that means men are more likely to burn off the calories they consume even without any exercise.

- *Age.* You know how little kids seem to have boundless amounts of energy? Their bodies are fresh and supple and young—they're constantly burning calories. However, as we age, our bodies tend to lose muscle mass, and this slows down our BMR. Therefore, we tend to accumulate more fat as we get older.

- *Body build.* Do you have a very muscular frame, or do you carry a lot of fat? Predictably, the people with lots of muscles have higher BMRs than do the people with lots of fat.

In fact, let's run through a hypothetical situation. Take a young man in his early twenties who exercises a lot. His build is very athletic, so what would you expect his BMR to be? Pretty high, right? Of course. Like I said, he's young, he's male, his build is lean, meaning muscular instead of fatty. He falls into all the optimum BMR categories. Therefore his metabolism is probably high. In fact, it works overtime, burning off his calories even when he's at rest.

Here's an interesting fact you should know: According to the Mayo Clinic, *our BMRs can account for burning up to 75 percent of the calories we consume.* Seventy-five percent! That means our bodies can burn up to three-quarters of our daily calorie intake simply by breathing, circulating blood, replacing cells, and so on.

But wait, it gets better. *Our bodies can burn off an additional 10 percent or so as they work to turn food into energy.* With all those calories being burned, how can anyone ever get fat? (That's a trick question, of course. You and I know the answer to that.)

So now let's take another example: a woman in her late sixties who's always tended toward pudgy. She doesn't get out and exercise; instead she leads a sedentary life. What would you expect her BMR to be? You got it. Probably pretty low. She's of a certain age and she's female (on the BMR scale, that's two strikes against) and she isn't working to build up the muscles that keep burning fat all the time.

I'll repeat this again before we continue, as it's very, very important: *Muscles have the power to burn calories even after you've stopped exercising.*

Therefore, to get fit, we want to build muscles. And to build muscles, we have to begin a simple course of strength training. In everyday terms, this means we should start lifting weights.

Now hang on a second. I understand that I may have just turned some people off, but you've probably got the wrong idea. We've all seen the Hans and Franz skit from *Saturday Night Live*. You know the one I'm talking about: Two big, muscle-bound guys keep saying, "We are here to *pump you up!*" And then they start flexing to beat the band.

Yes, there are people who spend their whole lives sculpting muscles most human beings don't even know they possess. But let me be clear: I'm not asking you to train so you can bench-press an Oldsmobile. I'm simply saying this:

> *To get fit, you should learn some basic strength-training*
> *exercises and build them into your routine. If you do that,*
> *you'll gain muscle. Gaining muscle burns more calories,*
> *which helps you burn more fat. Which helps you get more fit.*

By the way, as an added benefit, strength-training also improves your balance. Yes, that's another twofer for those of you who are paying attention.

And you don't have to join a gym. A simple set of dumbbells can be purchased at any sporting goods store. Frankly, you don't even have to buy a *complete* set of dumbbells. Start with one if that's all you can do. Hold it in one hand, do your routine, then pass it off to your other hand and do your routine on that side.

So how does weight training help you get fit? We already know that aerobic exercises help us lose weight. We walk, we bike, we swim, we run, we dance, and whenever we do these things, our heart rates increase and our muscles work hard and end up consuming more oxygen. Therefore they burn off more calories and our excess pounds just melt away.

But what happens when we stop performing aerobic exercise? Generally speaking, our bodies' heightened metabolisms will revert to their pre-exercise levels within about half an hour. Put differently, our bodies will still burn calories as if we're exercising up to thirty minutes after we've stopped. That's pretty good, right? You get thirty minutes of calorie burning for free. But why stop there? *If you're very muscular, you can multiply that thirty minutes times four.*

There's a very interesting study that was published in 2001 in a journal called *Medicine and Science in Sports and Exercise.* Researchers at Johns Hopkins and Arizona State Universities found that muscle tissue developed by weight training (sometimes called "resistance training") *can prolong the increased calorie burn of aerobic exercise for up to two hours after the exercise has stopped.*[25]

In other words, being more muscular can pay huge dividends in our efforts to lose weight. Far and above our BMR, muscular people can keep burning calories up to four times longer than "not-so-muscular" people can after exercise has stopped. Therefore, the more muscles we have, the more calories we burn in this post-exercise state. Which means we can shed pounds while watching a movie or reading a book. We can go for a walk with friends or spend time with our families and the pounds are still melting away. Our muscles' capacity for "prolonged burn" is an amazing phenomenon, and tremendously useful as we work to get fit.

So how much muscle weight should you gain? That's basically up to you. By now, I'm sure you can predict my feelings on the matter. I'm not advocating that you take a lot of whey protein supplements and bulk up to the point where you can beat Arnold Schwarzenegger in a bout of arm wrestling. *Remember that muscle tissue has its own weight. The more we put on, the heavier we are.* The only difference is that muscle weight is lean weight. Healthy weight. So I recommend that you shoot for a balance.

Can you lose weight without starting a light regimen of resistance training? Sure you can. I know I did. I didn't start lifting weights until a year or two after leaving Duke. But make no mistake: *You'll derive the maximum benefit from your aerobic workouts by adding a bit of weight training.*

Fit Tip #17: Manage Your Expectations
(Check Back in with Your Inspiration)

I get it. Exercise can be daunting to some, especially when you're just starting out (I know that's how it was for me). But here's a tip that can remedy that: *Change your expectations.*

A lot of people watch football, for instance (go with me on this tangent). And why shouldn't we? Football's a popular sport. But sometimes we see these guys running around at mach 3 on a gridiron, leaping into the air like gazelles, and slamming into each other head-first and we think: *Aha!* That's *what I call being in shape. I'll never be like that!*

Well, okay. You're probably right. But don't do yourself this massive disservice. *Stop comparing yourself to people who've made being fit their career.* In fact, stop comparing yourself to anyone but yourself. There's a wonderful line in the poem *Desiderata*: "If you compare yourself with others, you may become vain and bitter, for always there will be greater and lesser persons than yourself." That's a nice way of saying, "Who cares what other people are doing or thinking?" You're lucky. You've got plenty of things to work on for the moment. Best to focus on that. If you do, you might be surprised. You just might love the results.

Changing your expectations very often means:

- Slowing down

- Remembering to take things one at a time. This isn't a sprint, it's forever.

- Refusing to compare yourself to the progress of other people

- Focusing on the goals you've set for yourself

- Remembering that real fitness is a lifelong goal, not a victory of moments

- Looking forward to the next small goal you've set for yourself

If you're having one of those days when you just can't seem to muster the courage to stick to your routine or go for your walk or pick up the dumbbells and lift a few weights, I suggest that you take a moment, sit down, and hold a meeting with yourself. Touch base with why you wanted to get fit in the first place.

Was it because you wanted to reclaim your pride? Did you finally get so fed up with yourself that you realized you deserve more out of life? That's a very positive motivation, but negative ones can work just as well. Did your doctor sit you down and outline the grim possibilities you faced if you stayed heavy? Did you have a big scare? (I know I did—you're not alone on that one.)

Are you concerned about the strain you're causing on your family and friends? *Very often, doing things for other people's sake can provide a very powerful motivation.* What does your being fit mean to the people who are closest to you? Does it mean that you'll be able to dance with your daughter on her wedding day? Take your son on a camping trip? Have a great time with your partner on vacation? Insert any goal you want here (and, yes, I used the word "goal" on purpose). If you're getting fit for someone else, you can use that as your key inspiration.

Whatever the reason or reasons you have, check in with them now and then. Sit down with yourself. Revisit your motivations and be honest with yourself. *Because that first inspiration is you at your finest, the power source in your quest to get fit.*

Small goals are the way to go. *Setting and meeting small, reasonable goals can pave the road to bliss.* Is this kind of talk starting to sound familiar? Good. If it does, you're coming along.

Ultimately, I hope that getting fit means this: *You're keeping your body in shape to take advantage of all the wonderful opportunities that life so often throws our way.* If that's the expectation you have, you can exercise practically anywhere, or at any time. Your habits can be flexible to serve your ultimate goal, and you can pursue fitness in a way that's personal to you: your needs, your druthers, your resources, your schedule.

In fact, now that we're on the subject of personalizing a fitness routine, I offer this next Fit Tip. It's a very important recommendation for people whose schedules disallow consistent routines. It also applies to those days that get so hectic, so out of hand, that you just can't get your workout in. And for anyone who doesn't go to a gym (for whatever reason), it presents alternatives to traditional exercise. This important Fit Tip is:

Fit Tip #18: A Body in Motion Stays in Motion (Build Exercise into Your Daily Tasks)

Here's a scenario that may come up. I call it the Hectic Day at Work. Your first meeting starts at 8 a.m. sharp. Try as you might, you just can't get up that morning at six o'clock to hit the gym like you usually do. And that first meeting is just the beginning. The rest of your morning is booked solid with more meetings and presentations. Lunch is a meeting with a new client. The afternoon turns into an awful campaign of putting out fires as more fires pop up. You don't get home until 8 p.m., and then you're looking at a briefcase full of paperwork that *has* to be done by the very next morning so you can start the whole process all over again.

Suddenly, your fitness goals have jumped out the window, right? Suddenly, your health goes on the back burner. Correct?

Wrong. Days like this can happen to everyone at anytime. In other words, it doesn't matter what your profession is or how well you've planned your schedule or how heavily you've prioritized your quest to get fit. Once in a while a day or two or even a week comes along and demands your attention.

Remember: That's okay. Do not get discouraged. Keep in mind, we're in this for the long haul, and detours occur on any long journey. In fact, detours often present some of the most interesting opportunities to get creative and stick to our goals in ways we never would have otherwise foreseen.

For instance, how will you eat on your Hectic Day at Work? By now we know that we must grab breakfast, even if it means having to improvise. If breakfast is just a piece of fruit we grab on the go, that's good. Better a piece of fruit in our stomachs than nothing in there at all.

By now, my more creative readers may have already stocked their purses and briefcases with snacks they know are healthy for them. You know. Just in case. They may have already figured out which vending machines or nearby stores stock little bags of unsalted pretzels or nuts or trail mix and so on. And they know how to handle themselves when they're out to eat at that client lunch. In short, they can adapt to even the craziest conditions and make sure that they're consuming good food. Also that they're jotting everything they eat down in their food journals. In other words, they're sticking to the goals they've set for themselves.

Okay, so that's how you'll handle eating on this truly challenging day. But what about exercise? How can you get your heart and lungs pumping during a day like this?

Isaac Newton gave us the answer. Remember his first law of physics? *A body in motion tends to stay in motion.* That body, of course, is you, and it's time we discussed all the ways that you can stay in motion without slipping into your gym clothes and putting in a traditional workout.

For instance, why are you taking the elevator if your office is on the fourth floor? I'm serious—what's wrong with the stairs? I'm sure your building has them, right? Great. Walk through the lobby, bypass the elevator, head for the stairwell. Pull open the door. Walk up the stairs to get to your office. Walk down them when you leave the building. Exercise can be simple as that, and you've built it into your day.

But wait a minute! you might be saying. *That's not* really *a workout!* Well, yes. In fact, it most certainly is. Where do you think they got the idea for all those StairMaster machines?

Just so I'm clear: These are not what I'd consider optimal conditions for exercise. Frankly, I think we'd both be happier if we could get to the gym or hit the street or that path in the park and swing into our normal routine. But we can't today; that's a fact of life. Okay, so what? We're not going to waste any time crying about it. Instead, we're going to do what we can. Get creative. Adapt.

The funny thing about stairs is that we find them practically every-where. They're all around us, in almost every building, just sitting there, waiting for someone to climb them. Most anyone can build climbing a few flights of stairs directly into a normal routine. I try to do it when-ever I can. Taking the stairs is a great way to keep your metabolism up throughout the day. As a bonus, it's also a great way to avoid annoying elevator Muzak.

Sure, you're not running a marathon here, you're just walking up four flights of stairs! It's tempting to think this won't make any differ-ence. But wait, you're coming back down again, right? Of course you are, eventually. Four flights up and four flights down. There. You see? That's *eight* flights of stairs.

But wait! What happens when you go out to lunch, looking forward to a nice hearty salad? Here's another occasion when you have to walk downstairs, then back up. That's sixteen flights of stairs! Did you know that the Empire State Building is eighty-five stories tall? It's true. Which means that you just walked one-fifth of the way up the Empire State Building—and it's only the middle of the day.

I want you to be aware of some very interesting studies. Researchers have already charted the effects that small doses of vigorous exercise (like stairs) can have on people who were otherwise considered sedentary. The results may shock you. *For people who've never exercised before, even a few flights of stairs a day can improve cardiovascular health.* But a group of British researchers took this concept one step further. They wanted to know how short the bouts of exercise could be while still providing health benefits. Again, the results may shock you.

A British team made a study of twenty-two college-aged women whose profile was considered "sedentary." Each woman was asked to walk up 199 steps, and to do so at a "brisk but comfortable pace." On average, while performing the exercise, the women's heart rates rose to 90 percent of their predicted maximum rate. That's pretty good exercise!

The women performed the exercise once per day the first week, but this number increased until, by the sixth and seventh weeks, they were ascending the stairs six times per day. By the end of the study, this modest, easy-to-implement exercise program saw the students more fit overall. Specifically, by the end of the study, their heart rates, oxygen intake, and blood lactate levels had all greatly reduced. In other words, the climb was not so hard anymore. Their bodies had adapted.[26]

Also, the women saw noticeable increases in their HDL (high-density lipoprotein) or "good" cholesterol levels. HDL works to scour the walls of our blood vessels, clearing away deposits of excess cholesterol (plaque) that can lead to heart attacks and strokes. The higher our HDL count goes, the more we're scrubbing our blood vessels clean, and exercise is one of the keys to making that happen. And yes, that includes even modest forms of exercise. Like climbing stairs.

I once heard of a man who traveled a lot for business. On each of these trips, his schedule was always jam-packed, but he didn't let that stop him. Each morning, he would roll out of bed and hit the floor and do a few pushups and sit-ups. Then, in the bathroom of his hotel room, he would use the sink as a balancing beam and do a series of slow squats and lunges to work the muscles of his lower body. Squats and lunges are great ways to build up leg and postural muscles. *Slow* squats and lunges really push us to develop strength, but also a great deal of balance.

This guy also found himself with ten minutes to kill at two different points in the day. Guess what he did with them? That's right. He couldn't really leave the hotel where all of his meetings were scheduled, but he spent those ten minutes walking around. That way, by the end of the day, he was able to write down "Walked twenty minutes" in his exercise journal. Along the way, he also got a really great feel for the hotel he was staying in—call that a bonus. And here's the part that blows me away. He repeated his series of squats and lunges when he got back to his room that evening. He also did another round of pushups and sit-ups before turning in for the night. Of course he wrote these exercises down in his journal, as well.

Again, are these ideal conditions? Probably not. But let's not fool ourselves. The day I've just described to you is full of activity. I have no doubt this gentleman's metabolism was moving along at a pretty good pace all day long. And here's the most important part: Everything I've mentioned so far—pushups, sit-ups, lunges, squats—requires no weights, no gym, no equipment. Just gravity and the weight of our bodies and (most importantly) the will to do the exercise.

But you've already got the will, right? Fantastic. And now you've found the way. When you're really committed to getting fit, nothing can stop you from reaching your goals. There are no obstacles, only challenges.

That being said, it's probably time for me to mention this next and very important point. It's one that I've had to remember and put into action now and again. When life gets rough, you need to remember:

Fit Tip #19: Be Gentle with Yourself

I have to mention this since we're being completely honest with each other. Situations come up in life that will knock us off our games. The sudden death of a loved one, for instance, provides a classic example, and one I can certainly speak to.

In 1996, my sister Christine died in a waterskiing accident. I was devastated beyond words. My mother had passed away in the earlier part of 1993, so now it was just my dad and me. Christine had been such a lively person, we found ourselves empty in her absence. Maybe you've been through something like this, or maybe you can imagine it. The feeling that overwhelmed me was one of tremendous disorientation, and that was during the better times. Most days, I felt nothing at all but a very peculiar numbness.

Devastated, my father and I committed ourselves to the ancient routine of taking calls and making arrangements. We accepted condolences from family and friends. You sort of feel like you're sleepwalking through the whole ordeal. *This isn't real*, you catch yourself thinking. *This is just an awfully bad dream, and one that will go away the moment I open my eyes.* But it doesn't.

I can tell you from firsthand experience: There's a natural inclination for people to eat in times of stress. But this time, there was a vital difference.

When my mom passed away, I hadn't yet gone to Duke, hadn't yet redefined the reasons why I ate what I did, which foods were healthy, and which were not. In 1993, all that work lay ahead of me. So I weathered my mother's passing by eating some pretty awful foods. Pizza and cookies and that sort of thing. I gorged myself on comfort food, because that's what I thought I needed right then. Junk food was giving me comfort.

Now compare that moment to three years later, when Chris died. That event was equally devastating, but I was able to get through it because, by that point, I had been to Duke. I had learned how to eat to nourish myself. So I wasn't about to eat pizza. By then, I knew how foods like that could affect me, and knew I preferred to steer clear. And yes, of course I still needed comfort. But junk food wouldn't give me that. Eating something healthy would. Taking care of myself would. This time, I got through a very bad stretch by leaning on my lifestyle.

Now let me make this point so it's clear: Even if I had eaten bad food, *that would have been completely okay.* And this is the point I'm trying to make:

> *Traumatic experiences challenge us. They challenge our lifestyle commitments but they don't spell complete disaster. Nothing ever does that because our lifestyles never end.*

So what exactly happened when Chris died? Yes, I fell out of my normal exercise routine. So what? I wasn't going to go to the gym on the day of my sister's funeral. And yes, I stopped keeping my food diary for a few weeks. Again: So what? It didn't matter. By that point, I knew my routine very well, and I certainly didn't need my food journal to remind me not to eat unhealthy food.

I may not have had the same level of discipline while I was grieving, but I wasn't backsliding. I may not have been sticking to my 1,500-calorie-a-day target, but I wasn't reaching for food as a knee-jerk reaction to grief. I wasn't eating a box of donuts. I wasn't eating pizza and cookies the way I had done back in '93. *I pretty much kept to my basic plan. I still made healthy meal choices. If I wasn't at the peak of my form, well . . . that was understandable.*

It took me a few days to get myself back on track. Eating healthy. Exercising. Writing things down. If I gained any weight, I figured, so what? No real damage was done. The whole point of lifestyle work is that life happens, and life isn't always happy. That means it's a good idea to recognize that, when a family member dies or something similar happens, one of the things you're going to want to do is eat. You *can* eat, and you *should* eat. But you shouldn't brand yourself as having no discipline or copping out. You can't beat yourself up. If anything, it's a time for you to you to be gentle with yourself. Get through that bad time, whatever it is. Then look toward the future.

If anything, I credit my fitness lifestyle with helping me get through that very dark time. I've sometimes heard it said that keeping fit is like having money in the bank. You save and you save and you never withdraw. You let the dividends compound because you never know when you'll need them. The work I'd done since my first time at Duke had given me a strong foundation. So did the people who loved me the most, and often in unexpected ways.

For instance, I'll never forget Betsy Hilton, the sister of one of my dearest friends, Gary. Gary had died in 1994 so Betsy knew the pain I was in. She also knew how strongly I'd committed myself to a healthy lifestyle. So when Chris died, Betsy made a point to bring over a low-cheese, low-fat vegetable lasagna. I'll never forget Betsy Hilton for that. *She didn't just make food, she made food for me.*

Now here's a tip I can offer you that will actually *help* you be gentle with yourself. If you practice this next Fit Tip, I'll bet you won't find yourself feeling locked in, bound by a rigid routine. It's a simple rule of thumb, and it boils down to this:

Fit Tip #20: You Can Have It All, But You Can't Have It All at Once

Is it important to stay focused on the lifestyle we've chosen? Of course it is, and now you know why: *Because it never goes away.* That's part of the trap in Diet Thinking, and maybe a trap you used to catch yourself in again and again before you picked up this book.

You might have started a diet or a brand new fitness routine. Maybe you even kept at it for a few weeks or a few months. But then what happened? Did you catch yourself falling into moods where your thought process started to change? Could be. Did you start to catch yourself thinking, *Well, well, look at me! I've lost the weight. I look so good! Bring on that pound cake!*

Don't worry if you did. It's natural. It's normal. And here's even better news:

You can treat yourself now and again. But now and again isn't always.

This reminds me of a story I heard while I was at Duke. A woman who'd been at the DFC was doing everything right. She was sticking to her meal plan, exercising, and losing lots of weight. But she had a certain militant quality to the way she was going about her routine. Everyone noticed it.

She was doing so well losing weight, but she wasn't living a balanced lifestyle. A balanced lifestyle doesn't give up everything forever. Sweets and pizza and other things are still a part of life. It's about finding that balance. If you deny yourself everything you like, eventually you'll give in. We're human. And if you think that is somehow "falling off the wagon" you will define that cookie, that pizza, as failure. Instead, you should build these things—rarely—into your plan. It's about the next seventy years, not the next seventy pounds.

Eventually, one of the staffers took this woman aside and gave her a pretty unusual assignment. The staffer told her to go to the cookie store at the Northgate Mall in Durham, order a chocolate-chip cookie, and eat it. "And not just eat it," the staffer said. "I want you to *enjoy* it."

I bet you can already see the moral behind this story. This woman had become so set in her ways, so inflexible, so demanding of herself that her counselors got concerned. In essence, they were telling her, *Look. This isn't a sprint, it's a marathon. It's not a diet, it's a lifestyle, remember? You really have to ease up on yourself. Treat yourself a bit more gently. And that means giving yourself some perks. You know? A little treat here and there? It's nice to look forward to little delights. In the long run, they're what keep us going.*

So. For anyone who's been reading this book and thinking that Bill Baroni says you should never enjoy a cupcake again, or a piece of wedding cake, or a hamburger, or *insert your favorite treat here*—well. Think again. I'm setting the record straight right now: That's simply not the case, not if you're living your lifestyle correctly. You can, in fact you *must*, treat yourself now and then. The only thing you should keep in mind is that *now and then isn't every day.*

Let's put this to the test. In fact, let's make an argument for treating yourself to a chocolate-chip cookie *once a week! Gosh,* you might be saying. *Bill, is that even possible?* Of course it is. Let's do the math in the following hypothetical situation.

Suppose you've been living up to your lifestyle goals for two months. Your weight's coming down. Your energy's up. You're having the time of your life. You review your food diary and notice that you've stuck to a schedule of 1,500 calories a day the whole time (on average). And all the while you've been exercising, and dutifully noting each day's workout in the margin of your journal, right next to what you ate.

Congratulations! You're sticking to your plan, and what a big step that is! I'll bet you're already noticing how your body has started to change.

Now you want to reward yourself somehow. Because rewards make us want to do even better, right? Think of how you feel when you get a raise at your job or a commendation for doing something good for your community. Or think of how you feel when you help a total stranger with some problem and they smile and say thank you. It feels pretty good, right? So good that it makes you want to do it again, to keep at it. I might even go so far as to say: You want to make it a lifestyle. But what are the things that you really love? Should you give them up forever?

Let's say you decide that you absolutely love chocolate chip cookies. And you think that it might be nice to have one really good chocolate chip cookie per week. That would be wonderful, right? That would be heaven! But can you do that and still stay true to your goals? Well, let's see . . .

You sit down at home and work out the math and find that one chocolate chip cookie (the brand you prefer) has 200 calories. How would it affect your plan to eat just one of these cookies per week?

7 days a week multiplied by 1,500 calories = 10,500 calories, or your normal calorie intake

+ 1 chocolate chip cookie = 10,700 calories per week

Total percentage increase in calories = 1.9%

Can your lifestyle absorb a treat like that? Sure. I think it can. In this case, taking on 200 additional calories a week is justified, even desirable, if it keeps you excited about the goals you've set for yourself.

Now, we just talked about chocolate chip cookies, but remember: That was just the hypothetical situation I chose. Really, you could make the same argument for whatever treat you enjoy the most, so long as you approach the situation realistically, from an informed point of view. It's about finding a balance that works for you. It's about understanding that treating yourself to something you enjoy every once in a while is probably okay. Doing it every day? Probably not.

And while we're on this subject, be warned: *Once you get hooked on being fit, you may come to find that the best reward you can give yourself is sticking to your goals!* These days, I can honestly think of nothing I'd rather eat than a healthy meal that satisfies the lifestyle I've built for myself. That, to me, is a true reward, the best one I could hope for.

But this notion of treating yourself now and then really comes in handiest during some tricky situations. Take the holidays, for instance. For people who've pledged to watch their weight, the holidays kick up all sorts of challenges. Lots of personal issues boil up. *Should I have that piece of pie? Should I go for a second helping of turkey or brisket, ham or lasagna, duck or goose, or what have you?*

The answer is: It really depends. How is your lifestyle going?

I remember my first big holiday after leaving the DFC. It was Easter, a very important holiday for me since it was one of those times when my mom and I spent lots of time cooking together. For years, I've celebrated Easter by hosting a dinner for family and friends. I'm surrounded by my most loved ones. Typically, I'll serve lamb and ham, and my guests will bring lots of sides. There are vegetable dishes—corn and broccoli, salad and mashed potatoes. For dessert, there are plenty of cookies and cakes and homemade pies and candies. If a fat kid wants to fall off his wagon, this is the place to do it.

Remember, up until that point, I'd been counting every single calorie. But then I remembered something we'd been taught at Duke:

Holidays are important things. They're all about living. They're all about life. For me, Easter is an important day. So I decided to enjoy it.

The day after Easter is another day, I thought. I would get up and stick to my plan and eat my 1,500 calories. But again, that was tomorrow. Today, I would enjoy Easter with my family.

Do you see the difference?

- Diet Thinking would have me stress out over every piece of lamb.

- Lifestyle Thinking allowed me to focus on the long haul, and that meant giving myself the latitude to enjoy the holiday.

And you know what? By recognizing that Easter is a big holiday for me, I *was* sticking to a plan. I'd *planned* to go off my plan for a day. I knew I would eat more than 1,500 calories, and I did. Having one day when I don't stick to 1,500 calories? That's okay. Remember how I said that holidays are all about life? Well, part of the reason I wanted to lose weight in the first place . . . part of the reason I wanted to get fit . . . was to *enjoy* life! To *participate* in it! To be alive for the next *seventy* Easters.

When I went to bed that night, I knew where I'd be the very next morning. You got it: I would be back at the gym. Perhaps I'd fix a brown bag lunch, then jot down everything that I ate in my food journal, counting the calories.

In other words, *a day when I strayed from my normal routine was not such a frightening thing.* Like any good vacation, I could use the departure to recharge my internal batteries. That way I could hit the ground running the moment the holiday ended. I'd planned for it. I was fine the next day. My lifestyle routine had been tried and tested. It stood there, right where I'd left it, waiting for me to return and pick it back up. So that's what I did. I swung back into my normal routine and felt all the better for that.

Part of leading a healthy lifestyle is giving yourself permission to splurge now and then. Tell yourself, *Hey, you know what? It's Christmas. Or the High Holy Days.* Whatever you celebrate, tell yourself that your lifestyle's going to change for a while to accommodate the season. Remember that holidays signify life. We celebrate love and abundance and peace and sometimes a joyful excess. None of these match up to Diet Thinking, so go with the flow and have fun.

Picture the Diet Thinker at a holiday gathering. He won't stand for all the food on the table. Like the Chocolate Chip Cookie Woman from Duke, he tries to hold fast to rules that don't really stand a chance in light of the situation. They break the very first moment he tries to uphold them—how can they not? They're far too rigid and therefore fragile. They simply aren't destined to last.

Now picture our friendly Lifestyle Thinker having the time of his life. He loves his time with family and friends, and he keeps a watchful eye out on what he's eating at parties and dinners. Not critical, just watchful. Our hero, Mr. Lifestyle Thinker, helps himself to whatever he likes and finds that—even by treating himself—he's still pretty close to his normal plan. Once this holiday season has passed, he'll slide back into his normal routine. Not feeling guilty. Not feeling bad. Just eager to get back to work.

Here's another way to demonstrate this. Suppose you take a Diet Thinker who's planned out each and every meal to arrive at 1,500 calories a day. Really, I want you to think about that. Every day, this guy hits his mark: *1,500 . . . 1,500 . . . 1,500 . . . Yay!* But then a holiday rolls around. He goes to a party with colleagues and friends and—whoops! He's up to 2,500 that day! So the next day Captain Diet Thinker might try to restrict his intake. Yesterday, he went 1,000 calories over his normal allotment. So today, he'll try to balance that out by only consuming 500.

To Diet Thinkers, this plan makes sense. They're just making up for the difference, they think. Just evening out the score. But of course they miss the obvious point: This kind of math is impossible. It represents thinking that's grown too rigid. Eating like this means stuffing your body one day while you starve it to death the next. A program like this is doomed to fail, as will the body that sticks to it. This sort of plan ignores our bodies' most basic needs. No one on earth could stick to that. It simply isn't feasible.

On the other hand, suppose you have Mr. Lifestyle Thinker who's on the exact same plan. Every day, he's hitting his mark: *1,500 calories . . . 1,500 calories . . . 1,500 calories . . .* and so on. Mr. Lifestyle Thinker finds himself happy with the progress he's made.

But then that holiday rolls around. Mr. Lifestyle Thinker goes to a party accompanied by his colleagues and friends (maybe he works with Diet Thinker—the two of them probably know each other). And— whoops! Can you guess what happens next?

Mr. Lifestyle Thinker has a great time and takes in 2,500 calories, a thousand more than he's used to. But the very next morning, you know what he does? He shrugs it off and gets back to work. In essence, he's thinking like this:

Well, okay. Yesterday I had 1,000 calories too many. Normally, that would be something to avoid, but yesterday I treated myself because it was a holiday. I'm glad I had a great time with my friends. Such a great group of people! Today, we're right back on schedule and I look forward to hitting my marks.

Contrast this attitude with what Mr. Diet Thinker was probably thinking:

I didn't hit my usual mark yesterday. I didn't hit 1,500. That means I'm a failure. I knew I was. I've always been a failure.

Poor, poor Mr. Diet Thinker. If he only knew. Going out and celebrating with friends isn't failure. It's life. Slow and steady wins the race. There will be vacations, holidays, fêtes, tours, trips, funerals, good things, bad things, things in between. You don't lose weight and get healthier to ignore the good things in life.

So what can we do about it? Nothing. Just relax. Enjoy the ride and go with the flow. Be gentle. Let it be.

Keep your food journal up to date. Make sure to check it now and again during really turbulent times. Do the math and let it guide you. See how you're making out. If you notice you've splurged for the past four days, that's great! I hope that you had a great time; you probably deserved it. Now let yourself get back on track, but don't let your thinking get rigid.

By the way, a closing note on this. You can tap all the skills we've covered so far—all the other Fit Tips—to make sure you're making the most of life. Make sure that you're having it all. Are you going to a holiday party but want to stay on your plan? Wonderful! Call ahead and speak to your hosts. Tell them you'll bring a vegetable platter. Tell them you'll bring some gourmet coffee instead of a bottle of wine. If the food is served as an open buffet, that's great! Why sit down to one big meal when instead you can make small plates and munch throughout the night? Skip the eggnog someone offers you. Toast the New Year with water instead. Offer to drive someone home at the end of a wonderful, fun-filled evening. Better yet, take a nice long walk. That'll really help you digest.

Work your lifestyle. Guess what'll happen. The world will keep getting better and better!

Putting It All to the Test

I finished law school in the spring of 1998 and moved back to my hometown. A few years later, I ran for the State Assembly. At the time, the irony of what I was doing felt pleasantly overwhelming. Since you know a bit more about me now and how my quest to get fit got started, I'll bet you can understand why.

Sometimes I think that my weight was one of the chief reasons I went into politics in the first place. Meaning that, when I was fourteen years old, when I first volunteered at Congressman Chris Smith's office, the people there appreciated me, and I appreciated *being* appreciated. Apart from the love I got from my parents and my sister, the congressman's office was the healthiest environment that a kid like me could find. I threw myself into the work and rose through the ranks pretty fast. Would I have been so driven if I hadn't been so heavy? That's a very interesting question. Frankly? Probably not.

But fast forward. By now you know that I lost the weight. I went to law school. I was healthy. Worked out every day. I ran in 5K races pretty routinely. I had a great job that I liked. I had great friends. My life was going really well. And now I had a chance to run for the state legislature.

I'd always wanted to serve in the state assembly. And now I was ready to put myself out there, to really commit to the job of getting elected.

Here again, my fitness played a big part in my decision. Because, as part of getting elected to the legislature, I went around knocking on ten thousand doors. That's no exaggeration, by the way. I knocked on 10,809 doors. Yes, we counted, and yes, that took a very long time, but we ran a seven-day-a-week campaign. Basically, when I wasn't at work, I was out there pounding the pavement.

And you know what? I still worked out every day. I was still eating healthy. How did I do it? I reflected a lot on previous campaigns I'd run. By then I knew the pitfalls that can start to dominate your decisions whenever you aren't being careful. But I actually made my campaign work part of my physical fitness routine. We've already said that walking is good, that walking is very healthy. And let me give you a word to the wise: You do a lot of walking when you're knocking on ten thousand doors.

But along with this, I also practiced everything we've discussed. I always kept healthy snacks around. I drank a lot of water. I counted my calories. Kept my food journal. Everything that you already know.

Did it work? Of course it did. In fact, it worked in more ways than one. Sure, I stayed very healthy through another challenging time. But also, come November, I had won a seat in the State Assembly. Another dream of mine had come true.

Fit Tip #21: Focus on How You Want to Feel

During the race, my campaign manager, Bill Stepien, asked me to gather some old photos. "Things that show you as a kid," he said. "I'm putting together some literature and I thought it might be good to show how active you've always been. You know, playing in the soccer league and Little League baseball, that kind of thing. You're the hometown kid."

Aha, I thought. He had a point, but all the same, I cringed. By then, it had been eight years since I'd first attended the Duke DFC. I'd worked very hard to improve myself. I'd overhauled my lifestyle and lost over 130 pounds. My life was in a really good place. I loved the law firm I worked for and had a great boss there, David Norcross. My schedule allowed me time every day to work out. I would run through my lunch hour.

In other words, I had finally started enjoying life as a healthy person, a fit person. And the notion that everyone in my community would see pictures of me as a fat kid . . . well. Let's just say that idea held limited appeal for me.

But my campaign manager was smart. He stuck to his plan and kept asking me for the photos. I sighed and said okay, I'd start to look for them. Then I called dad and had him find some pictures of me as a kid.

He got me a bunch and I looked them over. There I was riding my bike at age ten. There I was playing T-ball. There I was getting in costume for Halloween. The high school play.

You know what? I thought. *I'm not* really *fat in these photos.* I mean, clearly I'm heavier than any of the other kids. But I'm not as heavy as I remember *feeling*. And that's when it hit me:

Fat is a state of mind. It's a belief system, that's all. And like every other belief system, it's completely self-perpetuating.

I felt fat, so I was fat.

I was fat, so I got fatter.

I believed I'd always be fat, so that's the way I was.

I believed I couldn't change, so I didn't.

Going to Duke that very first time broke the mold I had cast myself in. Or maybe that isn't precisely correct. Maybe it's more accurate to say that going to Duke taught me how to crack the mold, so I did. And that's what I started to focus on. Not breaking the mold. Not the mold being broken. That would be getting ahead of myself. I focused instead on that one little crack. Each morning when I got out of bed and drove to the Y. Each time I made my own brown bag lunch. Each time someone offered a beer or a glass of wine or a cocktail. I asked myself how I wanted to feel.

Fat or fit? Out of control or the guy in charge? Full of self-loathing or full of a deep and abiding self-respect?

When I put it like that, the answer was clear. And so shall it be for you.

> *Let go of any belief you might have that labels your fitness as sacrifice. That's focusing on the things that you've lost. Focus instead on what you have gained, and will always continue to gain by following your new lifestyle.*

Pay no attention to that fat kid in the rearview mirror. Focus instead on how you feel about this new life you've built for yourself. Imagine all the wonderful things you can do today, tomorrow, next week. Then move toward them.

Take the first step. You might be surprised. The rest might follow quite easily.

PART THREE:

FOR FAT KIDS AND THE PARENTS OF FAT KIDS

Obesity Is the Bubonic Plague
of the Twenty-first Century

I want you to think about history for a moment. During the Middle Ages (specifically between the years 1340 and 1350 AD), up to 60 percent of Europe's population was extinguished by something they called the Black Death. Most likely the Black Death was none other than the bubonic plague, a remarkably deadly disease that often gets carried by rodents and fleas.

The Black Death decimated Europe. In ten years' time, the world lost nearly a full quarter of its population to this one disease. It took 150 years to recover from the outbreak. To this day, Black Death could very well be the most deadly pandemic ever encountered by human civilization.

Until now.

The statistics on obesity in America terrify me. They indicate a national health crisis that rivals the bubonic plague, maybe even surpasses it. The scourge of obesity has already deeply dug its hooks into our population. We've started to suffer on so many levels: individually, economically, and socially. But that's not the worst part—not by far. I'm worried about our kids.

> *The obesity trend has worsened for years. It shows no sign of letting up, let alone of reversing itself. If we don't do something—and do something fast—our kids will inherit this awful disease that cripples the body and robs us all of our true potential in life.*

Of course some essential differences exist between modern Americans and people who suffered under the Black Death more than six hundred years ago. The biggest difference I can see is one that will have the most impact as we move to confront this disease. It's called knowledge, and the power of knowledge cannot be underestimated. I'll give you an example.

The people of medieval times knew practically nothing about the most rudimentary sanitation procedures. They didn't wash their hands before they ate or after they went to the bathroom. Often, they treated illnesses by applying leeches to a sick person's veins and sucking out their "polluted" blood. Or sometimes they went to the local barber, who opened a vein with a knife. What passed for knowledge during this era was little more than superstitious nonsense. I'd put more faith in one twenty-first century medical book than in all the greatest doctors and scientists medieval times could offer.

I'll say it again: Knowledge is power. Help stop this modern epidemic!

Here's what I find the most haunting. History tells us that the Black Death could have been contained quite easily. If people had figured out the disease was carried by fleas and rats, they could have altered their behaviors and kept themselves alive. The problem was lack of knowledge. For lack of knowledge, Europe fell.

Fast forward to the twenty-first century. Today, it's common knowledge that:

- Many Americans live unhealthy lives. This is not conjecture, it's fact. Anyone who needs further proof should go back to the start of this book and read the statistics again. Or pay attention to the news. Yes, obesity is a plague, and yes, it's spreading fast.

- An overweight and obese population strains the American health care system.

- Being overweight or obese takes a huge toll on our society. It hurts the economy, strains our family relationships, and robs us of the aspirations that we, as individuals, might otherwise attain.

- Public education comes up lacking with regard to issues of physical fitness.

- Federal, state, and local governments aren't doing everything they can to encourage citizens and industries to adopt healthy lifestyles.

And here's something that probably isn't considered common knowledge. *A child who is considered obese between the ages of ten and thirteen has an 80 percent likelihood of growing into an obese adult.*[27]

Okay. That's the bad news. And what does it amount to? Frankly, I think it's obvious. *It's time that we called ourselves to action. It's time to start fixing this problem together, and fast. Put simply, our future depends on it.*

But wait. I saved the best part for last. The best piece of knowledge, the one that might save us, boils down to this:

> *Getting fit for the rest of your life isn't an act of magic.*
> *Anyone can learn how to do it. The skills required are*
> *easily taught and easily learned, as well. Just about*
> *anyone can put them into practice, and fast. In fact, you*
> *can start today.*

In the next part of this book, I'm going to talk honestly about who's on your side (and who isn't) as you try to lose weight in America. If you're serious about getting fit, I think you'll appreciate that.

Most importantly, I'm going to talk about what to do if you have a child who's obese. This is a sensitive issue these days, but one that certainly needs to be handled (and handled effectively) to ensure your family's healthy future.

Some of the steps I'll recommend are simple to implement. Some of them are not. But you already knew that, didn't you? If you've already read this far in my book, I'll bet you're willing to hear me out. For your own sake or for the sake of your kids. Perhaps for the sake of us all.

The Forces Working against Your Child

'll tell you a secret that doctors know: Everyone—every human being—comes into the world with genetic predispositions. Some of us are prone to be tall. Some of us will start to lose our hair at a certain age. Some are gifted with excellent eyesight that age refuses to dim. Some of us don't seem to age at all. The years skip past and these people seem to stay the same, largely unchanged while others are not.

As with any other trait, some children can be genetically predisposed toward obesity. A child who has one overweight parent is much more likely to be overweight, as well. *However, if both parents are overweight, the child's chances of being overweight as well can be nearly double the norm.*[28] According to an article published by the *American Academy of Child & Adolescent Psychiatry*, if one parent is obese, a child has a 50 percent chance of being obese. But if both parents are obese, a child has an 80 percent chance of being obese.[29]

The exact causality of this relationship remains an open question. For instance, sometimes both parents are fat because they engage in unhealthy behaviors (poor eating habits, sedentary lifestyle, etc.). In this case, the child may be fat from copying these behaviors. This actually poses the best-case scenario. It means that no medical reason exists for the child to be overweight. It may require work, but the child, most likely, can learn to lead a healthier life. However, in cases where both parents are fat because of genetic predisposition, the child is more than likely fat from inheriting this same tendency.

But parents can play another key role in their children's lives by simply being aware of their child's actual weight, and knowing whether it falls within medical norms. One study shows that *parents who cannot or do not recognize their children as being at risk for being overweight stand a lesser chance of intervening. And this, in turn, results in an elevated risk of the children becoming obese. Which in turn elevates the children's risk of contracting any of the problems related to being obese.*[30]

Another critical factor to consider is a child's self-esteem. *Studies over the past twenty years indicate that overweight children have lower self-esteem than non-overweight children.* The difference isn't so massive as to cause any great alarm. In fact, as one researcher pointed out, "the degree of lowered self-esteem [among overweight children] is within the normal range for non-overweight children."

So okay, the problem is not in the numbers.[31] But what about the details?

Studies show that the way children perceive their bodies can often more accurately predict self-esteem issues than their actual body weights can. In other words, kids who are a few pounds overweight but feel they are fat (I refer you to Fit Tip #21) can develop depression as deep and disruptive as kids who are much heavier. Girls tend to get more depressed about their weight than boys do.[32]

Some studies pinpoint age eight as the most normal for the onset of weight-related self-esteem issues. And it may come as no surprise that incidents of peer discrimination against obese children run staggeringly high. In an age when incidents of bullying and the damage done by these incidents is dramatically on the rise, this last point should not be underestimated.

In fact, consider this: Remember at the beginning of this book when I said that most thin kids don't like having fat kids around? One study conducted in 1961 had ten- and eleven-year-old children review six images of other kids their age and arrange them in order of preference. The children in the study were asked, "Which of the children shown in the pictures would you most likely want to be friends with? Which would you least like to be friends with?"

The six pictures used in this study showed children who:

- were wheelchair bound

- were on crutches

- had an amputated hand

- possessed a facial disfigurement

- had average weight with no apparent disabilities, and

- were clearly overweight

The results of this study show that *children maintain a clear bias toward putting the overweight child last in their order of preference.* But perhaps even more shocking, the bias against the overweight child actually *widened* when the study was repeated forty-two years later in 2003.[33] If nothing else, this seems to reinforce the importance of parental guidance, nurturing, and compassion when dealing with children who have weight issues.

But regardless of how they feel about their weight, kids who are overweight or obese live lives of real and perpetual jeopardy. Apart from all the weight-inspired health problems I mentioned at the very beginning of this book, other, shocking examples exist of how being fat can inconvenience, discomfort, and sometimes literally kill a child.

One study conducted by the University of Missouri, Kansas City showed that the arterial walls of obese children very often resemble the arterial walls of forty-five-year-old adults who are prone to heart attacks and strokes.[34] Another study showed that obesity factors into about half of all pediatric gallstone cases.[35] Another showed that obese children carry increased risk of sleep apnea due to swollen tissues in their airways. Unable to get a full night's rest, these children sometimes develop behavioral problems because they're simply exhausted. To make matters worse, in some cases, the behavioral problems have been misdiagnosed as ADHD (attention deficit hyperactivity disorder). And doctors often treat ADHD with powerful medications. But in this case, the problem is not the child's brain. The problem is his or her weight.[36]

Unfortunately, I could go on and on, but you've probably already got the idea. Here's what I want you to take away from everything I've just said:

- There are genetic factors that indicate a child's propensity for obesity.

- So what? *Genetics don't predict everything.* A genetic predisposition to something simply creates different challenges.

- A lot of things that make a child fat equate to *environmental factors*, and these respond best to training and lifestyle, two points we'll talk about next.

Nowadays, the American Academy of Pediatrics "strongly encourages" pediatricians and health care providers to follow a three-point assessment scale in their clinical practices. To prevent childhood obesity, the clinician should:

- "Conduct thorough history including family history, eating, and physical activity with all patient's behaviors (including screen time, sweetened beverages, eating out, and fruits and vegetables).

- For each patient, consider patient's risk by virtue of family history, height and weight gain pattern, socioeconomic, ethnic, cultural, presence of comorbidities* and/or environmental factors.

- Beginning at age 2, calculate and plot BMI for all patients on a yearly basis."[37]

Please note how many of these factors you and I have already covered so far in this book (physical activity, sweetened beverages, eating out, etc.). And please note how seriously pediatricians are taking the issue of childhood obesity, how early they're starting to screen for it. "Beginning

---

Bill's note: Comorbidity is a medical term that indicates the presence of another disease or disorder in addition to a primary disease or disorder.

at age 2." I think this is a very smart practice. Frankly, children grow so quickly as well as in such unusual ways that it's often very hard to predict which child will have weight issues and which will not. A child who appears pudgy at age seven or eight might grow up to be a beanpole, while his willowy counterpart might start gaining pounds and not be able to keep them off. Best to keep tabs on both of these children early on and follow their development closely as they grow.

But the bottom line is this: *Check with your family doctor. Discuss your concerns and listen carefully to what he or she recommends. Let your doctor's advice form the backbone in your plan to battle your child's weight.*

And this, of course, is just the beginning. When confronting childhood obesity, it seems like the deck is stacked against us. Worst of all, the forces we might have thought were our allies often turn out to be culprits. I'm thinking now of our schools, which—sadly—have often left me underwhelmed by the way they prepare our children for fitness training. I'll tell you what I mean about that and let you be the judge.

The Battle with Soft Drinks

Schools that sell pizza and cupcakes for lunch. Vending machines stocked with sodas and candy. Our schools have become infested with poor nutritional options sold to children who gain weight by the day. Therefore it probably comes as no surprise that American public schools have come under fire for not doing enough to recognize and combat childhood obesity. Perhaps you've seen this in the news, or maybe you've even dealt with it within your local district.

I've heard some folks say, "Well, hey. This is America, right? Our schools should be able to sell whatever they want. This is a free market and choice is what it's all about."

On this particular matter, I disagree. In fact, I made it one of the very first issues I tackled once I got elected.

In 2005, when I was in the legislature, a bill was proposed to ban all sugared beverages in New Jersey public schools. Before a bill can become a law, it has go through an inquiry process. Back then, I sat as a member on the assembly's Education Committee. I was there when a lobbyist from one of the soda makers came in to testify. You can probably imagine what her stance was on the subject of banning sugared beverages from a very large consumer market, such as New Jersey's public schools.

The lobbyist sat before our committee and proceeded to tick off all the wonderful things that her company does to enhance community life. She noted how they offer plenty of drinks to suit healthier lifestyles, too. Water is one of their products, she said. She made sure to mention the brand by name. But it's all about choice, this lobbyist concluded. We should teach our kids to make choices in life instead of banning products outright. Then she said that no proven link exists between sugared sodas and childhood obesity.

I remember looking across at my fellow committee member, Bob Morgan. Bob was also new to the assembly, a pediatrician in his full time job. We looked at each other and I couldn't be certain which one of us was going to jump up first to refute this lobbyist's argument.

Essentially, her argument was that we need to allow people to make choices, a point with which, under most circumstances, I agree. But not when her argument extended to include that we should allow sugared sodas in schools because kids would make choices to drink them in the outside world, so why not in school?

My counter to that was simple. *A school is not the outside world.* For eight hours a day, we charge our public schools to educate our children as best we can. Why shouldn't that education also extend to what they're eating?

And as for the lobbyist's assertion that no proven link exists between sugared sodas and childhood obesity—well. I told her that just isn't true. In fact, before that hearing began, before the committee was tasked to vote, I had consulted two experts in the field.

One was Dr. Kelly Brownell, a professor of Psychology, Epidemiology, and Public Health at Yale University's Rudd Center for Food Policy and Obesity. Dr. Brownell's many publications include the book *Food Fight: The Inside Story of the Food Industry, America's Obesity Crisis, & What We Can Do About It.* His articles have been published in the *New York Times*, *Newsweek*, and the *New England Journal of Medicine.* His research has made him an internationally renowned expert in the fields of obesity and the intersection of behavior, environment, and health with public policy. In fact, in 2006, Dr. Brownell was named to *Time* magazine's list of "The World's 100 Most Influential People."

The other expert was Dr. Howard Eisenson, who currently serves as executive director of the Duke University Diet & Fitness Center. Dr. Eisenson graduated from Duke University Medical School and is considered a foremost expert on obesity, physical fitness, and promoting healthy behavior change in the fields of diet and exercise. He co-authored the book *The Duke Diet* with Dr. Martin Binks. He was kind enough to write the foreword to this book.

I explained to both of these experts—Dr. Eisenson and Dr. Brownell—the issue that stood before our committee. I asked them about any potential links that might exist between unhealthy children and soft drinks. Both doctors assured me that a direct link exists between sugared drinks and childhood obesity.

The lobbyist tried to cut me off, but I wasn't about to let her. I posed a hypothetical example of my own. Suppose a kid comes to school and starts using swear words, I said. Or terrible grammar. Suppose the student behaves disruptively. We'd correct that, right? Of course we would. And why? That's simple. Because schools have standards for that sort of thing, and these standards have to be upheld if the school is to be considered worth anything.

The lobbyist kept repeating the word *choice*, as if it were some kind of mantra. I said that I didn't think choice was the issue in this particular instance. Two plus two equals four in school. We don't let kids make a choice about that. We teach them what's proven, we teach them what's right. And that should extend to their health, as well. A school should lead by example.

Do we sell drugs in our schools? Of course not. That's something we punish. Do we sell alcohol in schools? Of course not. Apart from being illegal that would be grossly irresponsible. So why would we sell any other items we know can make children unhealthy? And don't give me any guff about how there's no proven link between sugared beverages and childhood obesity. That simply defies common sense. Healthier beverage choices abound, and these should gain our patronage.

Well. The lobbyist didn't seem very pleased. Our committee passed the bill to ban sugared beverages—passed it unanimously, I might add. And eventually, that bill became a law that would make the children in New Jersey public schools healthier.[38]

Walk the Talk

Over the past ten years or so, I've been invited to speak on the subject of fitness and healthy eating at many public schools. If possible, before the big day arrives, I like to hop on the Web and download a menu from the school at which I'll be speaking. Can you guess what I find? I'll bet that you can. Some of these menus seem to go out of their way to skirt nutritious options altogether. But one example really sticks in my mind. Let's call it the menu for Public School X.

The menu for Public School X had a note at the very bottom along with a cheerful-looking logo. The logo said that this note was something called a "Good Health Tip!" Note the exclamation point. Clearly, whoever wrote this menu must have thought that Good Health Tips! were really vital and exciting. You might imagine how interested I was to read it.

"Eat celery!" proclaimed the Good Health Tip! "Celery produces negative calories!"

Which is true, by the way. Celery is so tough and fibrous, it takes the human body more energy to digest it than the celery offers in calorie content. But then I checked the school's menu and guess what? Not one item on it featured celery. *Not one!*

Pork roll laced with sodium nitrate? Check. Hot dogs (another heavily processed pork product)? Check. Items with gobs and gobs of cheese? Check.

Vegetables? Er . . . no. Not really. Do french fries count? There were lots of french fries.

Desserts? Yup, all present and accounted for.

Wow, I thought. *What a useful tip*. And it is, but the menu hadn't followed through. If you're going to educate kids about food and you're saying that celery's healthy to eat . . . shouldn't you be offering some? Doesn't that sort of make sense?

We *must* serve healthier food in schools. But it's not just school cafeterias that are negligent. Many physical education departments are taking what I consider a totally wrong approach to teaching our kids how their bodies work.

Think back to your days in gym class. Did your teachers have you play games like crab soccer? Dodge ball? Steal the bacon? Duck, duck, goose? I know mine did, especially during elementary and middle school. Games like that play a big part in the curriculum in most American school systems. And yes, they're fun. Yes, they're teaching community, sportsmanship, and fair play. But are they good for teaching any kind of lifelong fitness skills? Absolutely not.

I submit that these games are just make-work for students. We could be using the time more effectively, teaching fun, socializing, and interesting games that also train our children to care for their bodies long-term. This kind of curriculum isn't hard to teach, and you can start as early as possible. But first we must change how we think.

Now don't get me wrong. A number of school systems around the country have already moved to this kind of cutting-edge approach to fitness education. They get students into the gym and teach them how to lift weights, for instance, as well as how to exercise aerobically in ways that are fun and deeply gratifying while also instilling the value of competition and hard work. But it's not enough. Given the extent of the American obesity crisis, we don't need a few isolated pockets of higher-minded fitness education. We need a revolution.

And by the way, please don't think I'm insisting that we turn every single student into a world class or even a competent athlete. Nor do I insist that for you. You don't have to play hockey like Wayne Gretzky or basketball like Michael Jordan or soccer like Brandi Chastain to be healthy. And no, I don't think it's the role of government to force physical fitness on anyone. But it's always been part of the American dream that excellent public education be made available to our children. Effective tools for lifelong physical fitness are certainly part of that. We have been remiss, I think, in not providing them.

It's time to take the long-term view. It's time to teach our children the value of Lifestyle Thinking, and start this as early as possible, so they can reap the maximum benefit.

Fit Tip #22: Eat Healthy, Eat as a Family

I know what you're probably thinking. *Yeah, right. Getting my family together these days is like herding cats. One child comes home every day after school and goes back out with his friends. Another one hits the books (she's the good one), but often her projects and late study groups obscure her evenings completely. My youngest one disappears to the basement to play his video games. One parent has to work late every night. The other one does all the household work—the cleaning, the laundry, the windows, the bills—and somehow that never leaves near enough time to cook decent meals for dinner. Besides, isn't that what takeout is for? The pizza guy's number is right on the fridge. He'll do all the work and he'll bring the meal here. I just have to answer the door . . .*

Believe me, I understand. Life can get busy—more so now than ever before. But that's not a decent excuse anymore. Why? Because you want to get fit. You want your kids to be fit. That's why you picked up this book, am I right? You're looking for solutions. Well, I've given you quite a few. Now it's time to lead by example. You have to start eating healthy and you have to eat as a family. There are two parts to that, so let's break them down. The first one you probably already know.

We've talked about eating healthy already. This whole book is full of tips about that. Am I saying you can't order pizza tonight? Well, no. I'm not saying that at all. Once in a while is totally fine, but no, you can't do it *all* the time. And whenever you order, you have to know how that pizza will fit with your lifestyle.

Remember the basic premise of weight loss. Calories in versus calories out. You want to lose weight? Okay, it's simple. Take fewer calories in. Or exercise more (that means calories out). Ideally, you should be doing both. Will slices of pizza work with your goals? Sure, I suppose every once in a while. We've already outlined procedures for splurging. *Yes, you can have it all, my friends, you just can't have it all at once.* Consider items like pizza a treat. Be wary of making them staples.

Let's look at the calorie breakdown on pizza. Admittedly, this is an inexact science since no two pizzas are ever the same. However, the basics I'm offering here should paint you a vivid picture. Let's say that you and your family like toppings: pepperoni and sausage. Assuming your pie has a regular crust, each slice will be 400 calories.

So how many slices comprise a meal? How many do you normally eat? Two? That's 800 calories, right? Three? Okay, that's 1,200. Once in a while, we've all seen people who pack away four or five slices, right? Go on. It's simple. Do the math. A way to get fit? Not really. I remember how I used to look forward to—how I loved—eating an entire pizza by myself. Now? I shudder at the thought.

So basically, pizza is not a good choice. It forces you to max out your calories all in one meal. For dinner, that means at the end of the day, when your body's digestion begins to slow down. Again, I'm not saying you can't eat pizza. I'm just saying you need to know the facts. Once you do, you can budget appropriately. Schedule times to enjoy it.

But let's look at this Fit Tip's second part, the part that says "Eat as a Family." Studies have shown that eating together can make a lasting effect on a child by forming lifelong eating habits trending toward the healthy.

One report conducted by the University of Minnesota studied 1,700 children when they were under the age of sixteen, and followed up with them five years later, after their twentieth birthdays. Interestingly, those who had eaten the majority of their meals with family reported making healthier food choices. Notably, they ate more fruits and vegetables, consumed fewer processed foods (including soft drinks), and generally consumed more essential nutrients such as magnesium, calcium, potassium, vitamin B6, and fiber.[39]

But those were just the breakdowns on the types of food consumed. The study showed encouraging data regarding behavioral choices. For instance, kids who grew up eating with family rarely skipped meals as adults, nor did they let themselves descend into unhealthy eating practices such as binge eating or excessive snacking. *In other words, kids who ate with their families learned good eating habits, then carried these habits forward into their lives as independent adults.*

Does that sound like something you'd want for your kids? Of course it is, but the study showed more, and the news gets better and better.

Let's take a look at one of the report's subsets. The study found that girls who regularly ate with their families are more likely to eat breakfast as adults. Combine this finding with plenty of research that shows that kids who tend to eat well-balanced breakfasts are much less likely to be overweight, to say nothing of being obese. Breakfast-eating children also tend to have higher cognitive skills in school, presumably since their brains are alert, well-fueled at the start of each day. Still other studies mark the trend that kids who share plenty of meals with their families tend to stick toward their optimum weight. They grow up with more enhanced awareness of food, as well as ways of preparing it to suit a healthy lifestyle.

So how does it work? How does having kids eat with their families instill healthier habits? Part of it has to do with parental oversight. Parents can watch their kids eat and offer instruction as needed. But really the key is socialization. Children look to adults in order to pattern specific behaviors. They pick up the good and they pick up the bad. If parents gripe about food, or gorge themselves, or make menu choices based on appetite rather than health and nourishment . . . well. Would it really come as a great surprise if their children followed suit?

By the way, the benefits of eating as a family extend far beyond your child's eating habits. Consider a study released in 2003 by the National Center on Addiction and Substance Abuse at Columbia University. Researchers there conducted a survey of 1,987 teenagers (a little more than half were boys) and 504 parents of teenagers across the forty-eight contiguous United States. In a nutshell, the study found that *teens who are more likely to eat dinner with their parents are less likely to drink alcohol, smoke, or use drugs. In fact, those teens that only ate dinner with their parents two nights a week or less doubled their risk of substance abuse.*[40]

Compare these findings to a study presented to the American Psychological Association in 1997. Dr. Blake Sperry Bowden and Dr. Jennie M. Zeisz classified more than five hundred teenagers as either "well-adjusted" or "not well-adjusted." For the purposes of the study, "well-adjusted" teens were those considered less likely to get depressed or use drugs, who demonstrated motivation toward school work, and who maintained good peer relationships. After breaking the teens into categories based on behavioral profiles, Bowden and Zeisz studied the number of times per week each teen ate dinner with his or her family. The numbers couldn't be clearer. On average, the well-adjusted teens ate dinner with their families five times a week. The not so well-adjusted teens? They averaged only three.

These studies go on and on. Some show that the presence of parents in a teenager's life before school, after school, at dinner, and bedtime significantly decreases outbursts of teenage rebellion. Others show increased testing scores for kids who eat with their families.

Am I going off on a tangent here? Frankly, I don't think so and I bet that you don't either. I bet that, if you're a parent, the most important thing in your life right now is the health and well-being of your child or children. You know the odds are stacked against them. You understand the distractions they face from peer pressure, video games, the Internet, and television. You know that your child's weight issue probably isn't a simple thing. Unless there's some medical issue at work, it probably has a lot less to do with food than it does with self-esteem and love and setting boundaries.

But nothing I've mentioned contradicts any of that. If anything, this tool I've presented—eat healthy, eat as a family—offers a means to solve several different problems at once. A fat kid is just the tip of the iceberg. And if the person reading this right now *is* a fat kid, then I ask you: Why did you pick up this book? What did you hope to get out of it? If you came to these pages looking for a plan to help you lose weight, if you wanted to find a way to start feeling better about yourself, then this is an excellent piece of advice: Start eating dinner with your family.

You don't have to do it every night (though clearly that would be best). But what about two nights a week? What about a Sunday brunch? What about cooking meals together so kids can see what goes into their food? What about cooking meals in advance and freezing them for later on, when schedules start to get tight?

This is the same as the Grocery Store Tour. This is the same as the Restaurant Experience. This is the same as preparing a healthy brown bag lunch every day. *Plan to eat, then eat your plan.* But this time, do it with family.

Fit Tip #23: Build a Support Group

Studies show that some form of weight loss counseling, when pursued alongside a healthy lifestyle plan, not only can help you shed unwanted pounds, but also plays a pivotal role in keeping those pounds off long-term. In fact, a very impressive piece of research offered by the National Weight Control Registry shows that people who lost weight and undertook a course of bimonthly support group meetings for one year were able to maintain their weight loss. Guess what happened to people who lost the weight and didn't go to some form of counseling? Yup. They put the weight back on, and typically more than half they'd lost.[41]

But notice that I said "*some form* of weight loss counseling." You don't have to lock yourself into something that feels uncomfortable. Having support can mean many things. It could mean taking sessions one-on-one with a licensed professional therapist, someone who's made it their specialty to analyze how their client's behaviors relate to and interact with food. It could mean a regular visit to Weight Watchers. For me, it means regular calls with my closest Duke friends.

But if, for whatever reason, none of these options works for you, fear not. Your weight loss counseling could take the form of something as simple as working with a "weight loss buddy." That's someone to whom you make a pledge and hold yourself accountable. Someone who, in turn, agrees to seek the same kind of support from you. Maybe you work out together. Maybe you talk openly about what you ate that day.

But wait! You might be thinking, *Hey, Bill! Isn't there some kind of corollary between Building a Support Group and Eating as a Family?*

If you think you've found a connection here, you're absolutely right. *Each of these Fit Tips revolves around sharing.* In fact, the core principle of these last two Fit Tips has to do with leveraging relationships and community to magnify the strength of your efforts and help you stick to your lifestyle goals. Put differently: *No one can do it alone.* And really, why would you want to?

We've already talked about how being overweight has become a national epidemic. And yes, this is horrible. Frightening and terrible. But believe it or not, there's a flip side to that. So many people are out there, right now, fighting the same good fight as you. *Imagine the massive support you'd feel if everyone in American who's trying to get fit was on your side for the lifelong haul!*

They are, by the way (and so am I). Right now you might not understand that. But very soon, I hope that you will. *Just like with anything else in life, true success most often comes the moment you surround yourself with a group or groups of like-minded people. People who support your goals.* That's why places like Duke exist, and that's why I'm writing this book for you.

I read a shocking study released by America on the Move, a nonprofit group that works to improve people's health and quality of life. Most everyone profiled in the study agreed it's invaluable to have the support of family and friends as you work to get fit. And yet, only a minuscule percentage of the same people surveyed said they'd received this kind of support. In other words, a disconnect exists. *We all know that getting the proper support will help us achieve and maintain our goals, but we also know that support is rare.*

Listen, I know how scary it is to open yourself up to another person or group of people about your weight issues. Remember, I was a fat kid for twenty-two years before I finally asked for help. And during those twenty-two years, I perfected every coping trick, every defense mechanism, and every emotional tactic to be found in the human psychological arsenal.

Being fat can hide sensitivities, fears, and insecurities. *When we start to lose weight, we strip away more than just unwanted pounds. We strip away parts of ourselves that we find no longer pertain to our goals.* And that can be a dizzying task, a rollercoaster ride for the soul. What better way to stay on course than to ask good friends to help navigate?

Seeking support is a type of commitment. I mention this because, by now, commitment is probably something you're used to. We made a commitment the first time we said, "Okay, from now on, I'll count calories." It was a commitment to vow, "Yes! From now on, I'll keep a food journal!" And it's certainly a commitment to say, "I know that I've been slacking off. From now on I'm going to take my health seriously, and that means a program of regular exercise."

But when it comes to seeking support from our peers, we sometimes catch ourselves thinking that this part of our lifestyle, this practice, this commitment to community isn't quite so important as, say, going to the gym. Don't fool yourself. It is. How many ways can I say this? *NO ONE WHO IS SUCCESSFUL DOES IT ALONE!*

I chose to support myself in a very powerful way by pledging to return to Duke for one week every year. This makes sense on a number of levels. In the first place, I've made such dear friends at Duke (and so many) that a trip back to the DFC gives me time to catch up with everyone. My friends and I meet for one week starting the first Sunday in July. We use our time together to laugh and joke and fill each other in on what's going on in our lives. We take some classes, exercise, eat healthy meals, and talk about all the goals we've accomplished over the past year. Over *all* the years.

People often ask me why I go back to Duke. Do I go back to work out? Sure. To eat healthy? Of course. But the truth is, I could do that at home. The real reason I go back to Duke is because of the people who've gone through all this with me—the people who, like you and me, are constantly struggling with their weight. We have something in common. Just like I assume people who battle other addictions do. We've gone through something together. And the importance of that cannot be overstated. It's the same reason I felt tremendously uncomfortable at the first fancy gym I tried to join when I first got back from Durham. The people there wouldn't understand. They wouldn't know where I was coming from.

My Duke friends and I can get very frank with each other. We confide in each other those nagging goals that we're having trouble obtaining. The obstacles we face. The hurdles and the challenges. We talk to each other about issues only fat people understand. Thin people are nice, but they haven't a clue the kinds of things we're dealing with. And we support each other, no matter what stage we're at in our individual practice. I have never felt more unconditional support than I have from the friends I have made at Duke. And I've never given that kind of support. That's important to note as well.

One Duke friend, Jane Berman, lives in South Florida. Jane has been very successful with her healthy Duke lifestyle while also working her way to being one of the top real estate brokers in the entire state. I know I can call Jane at any hour if I really need support and help. Stressful times? A brand new job? It doesn't matter. I know I can count on Jane and she will listen. She has been through more stresses in life than most people ever will and has come out stronger. She is one of the most important people in my life, and she reciprocates. Jane calls me when she needs someone to help.

Another friend is Marilyn Graber, a retired public schoolteacher from Rockville, Maryland, and truly one of the most amazing people I've ever met. She's loving, caring. She's got a great husband and two great kids and at one point she was going to die because she was obese. That's what brought her to Duke. Nowadays, she's come a long way. She speaks on the subject of living healthy. She's a great inspiration for me.

Ben Rippe owns a clothing store, a family business in Danville, Virginia. Susie Goldzman is another public schoolteacher from my home state of New Jersey. All of us are at different ages. With different professions. Different perspectives. From different parts of the country. Different life experiences.

It doesn't matter. We've all been through the same battle. In fact, we're fighting it as you read this. And that's why we can support each other. That's why I turn to these people first whenever I have a problem.

Frankly, these relationships are the greatest gift Duke gave me. Certainly, I consider them the most priceless. If I'm having a rough time, I know that I can call Janie Berman in the middle of the night and not only will she take the call, she'll have gone through something similar. These are the kinds of friendships where it doesn't matter how long it's been since the last time you saw one another. You're ready to pick up at any time. It's like riding a bike. You never forget. That's this group of people for me.

In the end, it's people who make our lives as rich as they can be. Money comes and money goes. So do houses, cars, clothes, jobs. Pretty much everything in our lives is ephemeral as the wind. But a good strong relationship? That's worth gold. The trust of another person? Platinum. Having someone pull for you when even you have started to stop? This is what really helps us lose weight. This is what really helps us get fit.

My Duke friends and I have all weathered challenges. We've weathered moments of self-doubt and setbacks and plateaus and holidays and the loss of loved ones. And that's why having those people on my journey is so important. Because they're people I can turn to and ask, "How did *you* get through that?" We share knowledge. We share tips. We talk to each other. Yes, we can share our emotions, sure. But we also share more practical things. Good strategies for living. Advice.

You need a support network for anything difficult you do in life. And as you and I know very well, getting fit and staying that way can be a difficult thing. Make it easier on yourself. Build your fitness support group. Seek out a discussion group. Go to your local hospital or fitness center. Almost every one runs programs to deal with various health issues, and weight is certainly one of them.

Find people who are like *us* and be with those people. Your Janes. Your Marilyns. Your Susies and your Bens. Listen to them. Spend time with them. Learn from them. And help them.

Common Sense in Society

On the subject of common sense, let's talk about government's recent efforts to legislate people's health. You've probably heard about the kinds of proposals I'm talking about. Many states and municipalities have already entertained them. The idea, in a nutshell, is that government—be it city, state, or federal—should impose a so-called "fat tax" on unhealthy foods, the same way it imposes a "vice tax" on goods like alcohol and tobacco. Proponents say that the money generated by these "fat taxes" will then go toward programs aimed at improving public health overall.

Now remember, I'm the guy who's been telling you all along to stay away from sodas and (some) processed foods. So you might be thinking, *Hang on, Bill. Wouldn't you* support *a fat tax?*

No, and here's why.

Taxes of this sort don't really help people lose weight. They just make food more expensive. Look, I understand the thinking that says, *We're trying to price unhealthy foods out of a certain market.* I also understand the thinking that says, *This means less people will be able to afford unhealthy foods. Which means less people will eat unhealthy foods. Which means less people will get fat. Which means the strain on the American health care system, the American workforce, our economy, and our families will start to abate.*

Sure, I understand this thinking. I simply don't agree with it. Everything I've outlined above boils down to nothing but theory.

Suppose you charge fifty bucks for a cheeseburger. Sure, you might keep some people from eating them. But raising the price by a small percentage? That just bleeds the public dry, and bleeding us dry won't help us get fit. It just makes a bad situation worse.

In my opinion, the answer lies with incentives, not with penalties. Reward, don't punish. Give people a tangible reason to stay fit and who knows? They just might surprise you.

For instance, a few years back the state of New Jersey created one of the dumbest public policy decisions I think has ever been made. (Don't worry if you're not from New Jersey, similar laws have since been passed in other states, as well.) The state levied a tax on gym memberships. The tax applied to monthly dues as well as initiation fees.

We're now penalizing people for trying to stay healthy!

The law was stupid. Dumb. Short-sighted. Dumb (did I say that?). Idiotic and counterproductive. I railed against it in the legislature. Over and over and over again. Eventually, the government partially repealed the tax. Not all the way and not enough. Essentially, it waived the tax for nonprofit establishments like YMCAs and JCCs and community recreation centers.

Still dumb if you ask my humble opinion. Still short-sighted and counterproductive. Because now they'd created a bias toward nonprofits over for-profit organizations. Hey, I'm a big fan of nonprofits; they serve a tremendous need in society. But you don't have to be a Nobel Prize–winning economist to know that pushing people away from competitive industry is never good for the economy.

Adding insult to injury, the amount of money collected by this tax was negligible at best. The state found itself with a budget shortfall and *voila!* Certain people started clamoring for new ways to close the gap, regardless of how effective they were (or weren't, as this case turned out to be).

It could be that such ridiculousness is another conversation for another time. But as far as your efforts to keep fit are concerned, I urge you: Keep your ear to the ground. Pay attention to public policy. Remember that you have a right to expect that the money you pay in taxes goes to improve your quality of life, not decrease it.

We shouldn't be taxing gym memberships. We should be moving to a taxation system at both a state and federal level that allows you to *deduct* your gym membership.

The reason we allow deductions for charitable contributions is that we *want* people to make those donations. Why? They make society better. When you donate to your local hospital charity, for instance, it makes the community better.

The same should go for gym memberships. By allowing people to deduct gym memberships from their taxes, we would provide an incentive for people to go to the gym, and therefore stay healthy. And that, in turn, would reduce the current strain on the health care system which stems from many problems, not the least of which is obesity.

Repeating the Past

These days, I'm not working out to lose weight. I'm not even working out to *maintain* my weight. I do it because I love how it feels. I love the energy. The endorphins. The rush. I do it because I learned to trade in the fake rush of donuts and junk food for something more exhilarating: a healthy lifestyle.

All my mistakes of eating badly and never exercising for all those years are memories, not current events. Now, in the full light of present day, I get to have a healthy, in-shape life because I broke out of the patterns that kept holding me back.

And so can you.

It isn't easy, that's for sure. But I learned that it's worth it.

A new lifestyle, one that looks beyond just dieting, toward a more colorful, meaningful life, is exactly what I got. And yes, I'll say it again. So can you.

Don't worry. Like I said before, you're not alone. Not hardly. I got fit, and so can you. If you can do it, so can we all. The *how* and the *why* and the *where* don't matter. The when, however, probably does. The when for you, I hope, is now. Today. This minute. Right now, while you're reading. This isn't a dream. It's real.

I won't say good-bye since this isn't the end. Remember, a lifestyle has no end. There's simply another day to keep living the life you've always wanted to lead.

Final thought: Being a Fat Kid makes me appreciate Getting Fit. And you will too.

ACKNOWLEDGMENTS

There are so many people who've played a part in the making of this book and the journey behind it. Thanks must go to my agent, Martha Kaplan, and my editor, Janice Goldklang, for all the advice and counsel that have made this book what it is. And that thanks extends to all the people at Globe Pequot whose contributions might not be apparent but surely have played key roles.

To my family, whose love and support on this journey are endless: My dad and June. The Curtin Family. The Ohio Baroni Family. The Censoplanos.

I am deeply indebted to the entire staff of the Duke University Diet & Fitness Center for all their hard work, dedication, and support. Because of them, I am alive to write this book. And of course this includes Dr. Howard Eisenson and his predecessor as director of the DFC, Dr. Michael Hamilton.

To my Duke group: Jane Berman. Marilyn Graber. Susan Goldzman. Ben Rippe. Jill Bloch. Michael Negreanu. Sue Evans. Mish Sutter. Anthony Rauseo. We are a group that is on this journey together—and I could not ask for a better, more loving group of people in my life.

My deepest love and thanks to all those who live this weight loss journey with me: my other families, the DiMarcos, the Linkimers, the Applelgets, and the Ballings. John and Cindy Holub. Michael and Gretchen DiMarco. Kristin Appelget. Sue Niederer. Todd Riffle. Matt Dowling.

To Andy and Mike: Thank you for making me realize how happy I can be by being exactly who I am.

Great thanks to the staff at the Hamilton YMCA and the Robert Wood Johnson University Hospital Center for Health & Wellness. They save lives every day.

Thanks to my staff and volunteers who worked so hard in my elections and my work in the Legislature.

And to the people of my hometown of Hamilton, New Jersey: Thanks for meeting me door to door and trusting me with your votes, hopes, and faith.

Fit Tips Quick Reference

Fat Foods and Their Approximate Calories

(Yes, you can eat them, but handle with care.)

Pizza

Cheese slice with regular crust	290
Cheese slice with pan-style crust	350
Pepperoni slice with regular crust	350
Pepperoni slice with pan-style crust	410
Sausage slice with regular crust	340
Sausage slice with pan-style crust	400

Fast Food

French toast sticks (serving of 5)	440
Chicken nuggets/tenders (8-piece)	350
Cheeseburger (6 oz.)	450
French fries (medium serving)	400
Onion rings (medium)	380
Mozzarella sticks (5 oz.)	470

Snacks

Potato chips (one small bag)	350
Soft pretzel (large)	480
Chocolate candy bar	280
Soft drink (16 oz. bottle)	200
Cheese nachos (100 grams)	300

Red Meat

Lean sirloin broiled, 4 oz.	210
Lean sirloin broiled, 6 oz.	320
Lean sirloin broiled, 8 oz.	430
Lean T-bone broiled, 4 oz.	200
Lean T-bone broiled, 6 oz.	300
Lean T-bone broiled, 8 oz.	400
Lean tenderloin broiled, 4 oz.	200
Lean tenderloin broiled, 6 oz.	305
Lean tenderloin broiled, 8 oz.	410

Other Entrees

Macaroni and cheese (1 cup)	400
Lasagna with meat sauce (10.5 oz.)	400
Chicken pot pie (7.5 oz.)	480
Baby back ribs (full rack)	1200+

Dessert Items

Apple pie (1 slice)	410
Pecan pie (1 slice)	500
Ice cream (1 cup)	260
Chocolate milk shake (16 oz.)	580
Vanilla milk shake (16 oz.)	550
Cheesecake (1 slice)	510
Jelly donut	290
Blueberry muffin	500
Croissant (plain)	320
Brownie (4-inch square)	400

Fit Foods and Their Approximate Calories

(Eat them! Enjoy them! They help you stay fit and taste fantastic, too!)

Breakfast Ideas

6 oz. cup of non-fat yogurt	80
1 cup of oatmeal, cooked	125
1 English muffin	120
1 banana, medium size	105
1 cup fresh blueberries	80
1 8 oz. glass of fresh orange juice	120
1 8 oz. glass of skim milk	80
Egg white omelet (4) with 1 cup fresh spinach leaves, diced onions, tomatoes, and mushrooms, plus herbs	130
1 slice whole grain toast	90

Chicken

4 oz. serving, boneless, skinless breast	110
6 oz. serving, boneless, skinless breast	137
8 oz. serving, boneless, skinless breast	164

Fish

6 oz. Atlantic salmon, cooked in dry heat	220
6 oz. smoked lox salmon	166
6 oz. tilapia, cooked in dry heat	150
6 oz. tuna steak, cooked in dry heat	180
4 oz. cod, baked or broiled	120

Seafood

4 oz. baked or broiled scallops	150
4 oz. steamed or broiled shrimp	115
3 oz. mussels cooked over dry heat	60

Pasta and Grains

1 slice multigrain or whole-wheat bread	90
$\frac{1}{2}$ cup pasta cooked (no butter, no oil)	100
$\frac{1}{2}$ cup pasta cooked (with $\frac{1}{4}$ cup marinara sauce)	140
$\frac{1}{2}$ cup cooked quinoa	130
$\frac{1}{2}$ cup cooked barley	120
$\frac{1}{2}$ cup brown rice	120

Nuts

$\frac{1}{2}$ cup dry roasted almonds	210
$\frac{1}{2}$ cup raw cashews	190
$\frac{1}{2}$ cup raw peanuts	210
$\frac{1}{2}$ cup raw walnuts	160

Beans and Legumes

$\frac{1}{2}$ cup cooked black beans	115
$\frac{1}{2}$ cup cooked garbanzo beans	140
$\frac{1}{2}$ cup cooked kidney beans	115
$\frac{1}{2}$ cup cooked lentils	115
$\frac{1}{2}$ cup cooked soybeans	150
4 oz. raw tofu	90
4 oz. cooked tempeh	220

Dairy

1 cup skim milk	80
1 cup 1% milk	100
$\frac{1}{2}$ cup fat-free cottage cheese	80

½ cup 2% milk fat cottage cheese	90
1 oz. part-skim mozzarella cheese	70
1 cup low-fat yogurt	155

Sides

1 small baked potato	130
1 medium baked potato	160
1 large baked potato	250 and up
½ cup steamed mixed vegetables	50
Small garden salad (no dressing)	50
1 cup minestrone soup	140
1 small ear of corn	60

Web Resources

Basal Metabolic Rate
www.bmi-calculator.net/bmr-calculator
Quickly calculate the number of calories you burn daily to satisfy your basal metabolic rate based on height, weight, age, and gender.

Body Mass Index
www.nhlbisupport.com/bmi
A site set up by the National Heart, Lung, and Blood Institute for calculating body mass index (BMI), or the measure of a person's body fat based on height and weight.

Calories Burned
www.mayoclinic.com/health/exercise/SM00109
With the understanding that the amount of calories each person burns during a specific activity can fluctuate, the Mayo Clinic nonetheless offers a good list of benchmarks per activity.

Calorie Counting
www.newcaloriecounter.com/articles/goverment/usda/usda_national_nutrient_database_for_standard_reference.html
According to the website, "The USDA National Nutrient Database for Standard Reference is one of the most comprehensive sources for evaluating the nutrient content of close to 8,000 food items. It is a major source of food composition used by both private and public sectors."

http://caloriecount.about.com/
A robust online community for people looking to count calories, and so much more. Membership is free and includes access to forums, articles, and computerized health tools. They even have a free iPhone app.

Childhood Obesity
www.cdc.gov/healthyyouth/obesity/facts.htm
The Centers for Disease Control and Prevention present the latest facts about childhood obesity, while presenting excellent resources on prevention and wellness.

www.mayoclinic.com/health/childhood-obesity/DS00698
The portal to the Mayo Clinic's online resources for recognizing and combating childhood obesity.

Healthy Cooking
http://allrecipes.com/Recipes/healthy-recipes/main.aspx
A searchable database listing close to two thousand recipes for every palate, with special categories for low calorie, low carb, low cholesterol, low fat, and low sodium foods, meals for diabetics, and many more.

www.heart.org/HEARTORG/GettingHealthy/NutritionCenter/ HealthyCooking/Healthy-Cooking_UCM_001183_SubHomePage .jsp
A comprehensive database of information on nutrition, recipes, and seasonal meal preparation, maintained by the American Heart Association.

Lifestyle Change
www.dukehealth.org/services/diet_and_fitness/about/
The website for the Duke University Diet & Fitness Center.

www.mayoclinic.com/health/weight-loss/HQ01625
A nice summary from the Mayo Clinic of six cornerstones of effective lifestyle change. Links to other important Mayo articles are included at the bottom of the page.

Obesity Definitions and Treatment
www.nhlbi.nih.gov/guidelines/obesity/prctgd_c.pdf
"The Practical Guide Identification, Evaluation, and Treatment of Overweight and Obesity in Adults" as published by the Obesity Education Initiative of the National Heart, Lung, and Blood Institute.

www.nlm.nih.gov/medlineplus/obesity.html
An excellent listing of articles, videos, and other resources maintained by the U.S. National Library of Medicine and the National Institutes of Health. This content is also available in Spanish, Arabic, and Vietnamese.

Physical Activity Guidelines
www.health.gov/paguidelines/
Guidelines on how to incorporate physical activity into your everyday routine, as put out by the U.S. Department of Health and Human Services.

www.cdc.gov/physicalactivity/everyone/guidelines/index.html
Guidelines under the heading "How Much Physical Activity Do You Need" put out by the Centers for Disease Control and Prevention. The information offered has been broken down into three age categories: Children (6 to 17 years old); Adults (18 to 64); and Older Adults (65 +).

Food Journal (Sample)

Date and Day:
10/4/11, Tuesday

Calorie Goal:
1700 calories

Meal	Food (Item + Amount)	Calories	Location	Mood	Notes
Breakfast	1 cup oatmeal 6 egg white omelet Vegetable side	160 50 15	at home	Great!	Big meeting today
Snack	Apple	55	at my desk in the office	Good	Meeting approaches
Lunch	Grilled Chicken Cobb salad	530	out with the team	Great	Meeting a success!
Snack	Yogurt pretzel snack pack	100	at my desk	Great	All good!
Dinner	6 oz. Atlantic salmon cooked dry heat 1/2 cup brown rice 1/2 cup kidney beans	220 120 115	home	Great	Good day!
Snack	1 cup ice cream	260	home	Great	Because I deserve a treat! I rock!
	Total Calories:	1625			

Exercise Journal (Sample)

Day	Activity	Amount of Time	Notes
Monday	Walk	30 min.	After dinner.
Tuesday	Walk	35 min.	That's 5 more minutes than I did yesterday!
Wednesday	Walk	35 min.	The new "35" feels good.
Thursday	Bike	40 min.	Great day for a ride in the park, figured I'd switch things up a bit.
Friday	Steps	20 flights	Raining outside so I put my headphones on and walked up and down the stairs 20 times before dinner. Tough!
Saturday	Walk	35 min.	Morning. Tried some new music today, felt good!
Sunday	Walk	35 min.	Morning. Might take a break tomorrow, but then I'll try walking 40 minutes!

ENDNOTES

1 Flegal, K. M.; Carroll, M. D.; Ogden, C. L.; Curtin, L. R.; "Prevalence and trends in obesity among US adults, 1999–2008." *The Journal of the American Medical Association* 2010; DOI: 10.1001/jama.2009.2014. Available at: www.jama.com. Also: Ogden, C. L.; Carroll, M. D.; Curtin L. R.; et al. "Prevalence of high body mass index in US children and adolescents, 2007–2008." *The Journal of the American Medical Association* 2010; DOI: 10.1001/jama.2009.2012. Available at: www.jama.com.

2 National Institutes of Health (National Heart, Lung, and Blood Institute in cooperation with the National Institute of Diabetes and Digestive Kidney Issues). "Clinical guidelines on the identification, evaluation, and treatment of overweight and obesity in adults." *The Evidence Report.* NIH Publication No. 98–4083, September 1998, National Institutes of Health. Available at: www.nhlbi.nih.gov/guidelines/obesity/ob_gdlns.pdf.

3 *New York Times* News Service. "Diabetes Cases Up. Experts Cite Obesity, Too Little Exercise." As appeared in the *Chicago Tribune.* August 4, 2000. Available at: http://articles.chicagotribune.com/2000-8-24/news/000824375_1_diabetes-care-diabetes-division-high-calorie-food.

4 Centers for Disease Control website article. "Overweight and Obesity: Economic Consequences." Date and author available at: www.cdc.gov/obesity/causes/economics.html.

5 Behan, Donald F.; Cox, Samuel H. Society of Actuaries, Committee on Life Insurance Research. "Obesity and Its Relation to Mortality and Morbidity Costs." December 2010. Available at: www.soa.org/files/pdf/research-2011-obesity-relation-mortality.pdf.

6 Zoroya, Gregg. "Pentagon reports U.S. troops obesity doubles since 2003." *USA Today,* article updated February 9, 2009. Available at: www.usatoday.com/news/military/2009-02-09-obesity_N.htm.

7 Ogden, Cynthia, Ph.D.; Carroll, Margaret, M.S.P.H. "Prevalence of Obesity Among Children and Adolescents: United States, Trends 1963–1965 Through 2007–2008." *Division of Health and Nutrition Examination Surveys.* June 2010. Available at: www.cdc.gov/nchs/data/hestat/obesity_child_07_08/obesity_child_07_08.pdf.

8 Ogden, C. L.; Flegal, Katherine M.; Carroll, Margaret D.; et al. "Prevalence of overweight and obesity in the United States, 1999–2004." *Journal of the American Medical Association.* 2006. Available at: http://jama.ama-assn.org/content/295/13/1549.full.pdf+html. Also: Ogden, C. L.; Flegal, Katherine M.; Carroll, Margaret D.; et al.

"Prevalence and trends in overweight among US children and adolescents, 1999–2000." *Journal of the American Medical Association.* 2002. Available at: http://jama.ama-assn .org/content/288/14/1723.full.

9   Cawley, John. "The economics of childhood obesity." *Health Affairs*, March 2010. Volume 29—Number 3. Available at: http://content.healthaffairs.org/content/ 29/3/364.abstract.

10   "The U.S. Weight Loss and Diet Control Market (9th edition)." LaRosa, John (with Goldstein, F.; Levine, R.; Spencer, T.; Colditz, G.A.; Stampfer, J. J. (MarketData Enterprises, Inc., 1996).

11   National Institutes of Health (National Heart, Lung, and Blood Institute), Vasan, Ramachandran, MD; Dhingra, Ravi, MD; et al. "Soft drink consumption and risk of developing cardio-metabolic risk factors and the metabolic syndrome in middle aged adults in the community, 2007." Posted online at *Circulation.* Available at: http://circ .ahajournals.org/cgi/content/short/CIRCULATIONAHA.107.689935v1.

12   Doheny, Kathleen. "Can diet soda boost your risk of stroke? Researchers find a 61% increased risk among those who drink daily." *U.S. News & World Report.* February 9, 2011. Available at: http://health.usnews.com/health-news/family-health/heart/ articles/2011/02/09/can-diet-soda-boost-your-stroke-risk.

13   ABC News (actual author uncited). "Caffeine Nation: Diet Coke Addiction. Consumers Spend More than $21 Billion on Diet Sodas Each Year," August 4, 2007. Available at: http://abcnews.go.com/GMA/PersonalBest/story?id=3447205&page=1.

14   Dufault, Renee; LeBlanc, Blaise; Schnoll, Roseanne; et al. "Mercury from chlor-alkali plants: measure concentrations in food product sugar." *Environmental Health.* January 2009. Volume 8—Number 2. Available at: www.ehjournal.net/content/8/1/2.

15   Robertson, Donald S., MD, M.Sc. *The Snowbird Diet: 12 Days to a Slender Future and a Lifetime of Gourmet Dining* (Warner Books, 1986).

16   "The Water in You" posted on the United States Geological Survey site. Available at: http://ga.water.usgs.gov/edu/propertyyou.html.

17   Mann, Traci; Tomiyama, Janet; et al. "Medicare's search for effective obesity treatments: Diets are not the answer." *American Psychologist.* April 2007. Volume 62—Number 3. Pages 220–233. Available at: http://psycnet.apa.org/journals/ amp/62/3/220/.

18   Hollis, Jack F., PhD; Gullion, Christina, M., PhD; Stevens, Victor J., PhD; et al. "Weight loss during the intensive intervention phase of the weight-loss maintenance trial." *American Journal of Preventive Medicine*, August 2008. Volume 35—Issue 2, Pages 118–126, Available at: www.ajpm-online.net/article/S0749-3797(08)00374-7/ abstract.

19   Bellisle, France; Dalix, Anne-Marie (From INSERM U341, Hôpital Hôtel-Dieu Paris). "Cognitive restraint can be offset by distraction, leading to increased meal intake in women." *American Journal of Clinical Nutrition*, August 2001. Volume 74, No 2, 197–200. Available at: www.ajcn.org/content/74/2/197.full.

20   Kaiser Permanente website article. "CHR Study Finds Keeping Food Diaries Double Weight Loss." July 2008. Author unknown. Available at: www.kpchr.org/ research/public/news.aspx?newsid=3. Offered as commentary to the following study, also by Kaiser Permanente: Hollis, Jack F., PhD; Gullion, Christina, M., PhD; Stevens, Victor J., PhD; et al. "Weight loss during the intensive intervention phase of the weight-loss maintenance trial." *American Journal of Preventive Medicine*, August 2008. Volume 35, Issue 2, Pages 118–126. Available at: www.ajpm-online.net/article/ S0749-3797(08)00374-7/abstract.

21   Rickman, Joy C.; Barrett, Diane M.; Bruhn, Christine M. "Nutritional comparison of fresh, frozen and canned fruits and vegetables. Part 1. Vitamins C and B and phenolic compounds." *Journal of the Science of Food and Agriculture*. 2007. Volume 87. Pages 930–944. Available at: www.letsgo.org/resources/5210/five/CannedAndFrozen Facts.pdf.

22   Jeffrey, Robert W.; Rydell, Sarah; Dunn, Caroline L.; et al. "Effects of portion size on chronic energy intake." *International Journal of Behavioral Nutrition and Physical Activity*, June 2007. Volume 4—Number 27. Available at: www.ijbnpa.org/content/4/1/27.

23   Sun, Weimin; Wang, Wei; Kim, Jung; et al. "Anti-Cancer Effect of Resveratrol Is Associated with Induction of Apoptosis via a Mitochondrial Pathway Alignment." *Advances in Experimental Medicine and Biology*, March 2008. Volume 614–Part IV. Pages. 179–186. Available at: https://springerlink3.metapress.com/content/ u012274485583434/resource-secured/?target=fulltext.pdf&sid=4m0cb4idelypis45ch0tz i3i&sh=springerlink.com.

24   See also: Mink, Pamela J.; Scrafford, Carolyn G.; Barraj, Leila M.; "Flavonoid intake and cardiovascular disease mortality: a prospective study in postmenopausal women." *American Journal of Clinical Nutrition*, March 2007. Volume 85—Number 3. Pages 895–909. Available at: www.ajcn.org/content/85/3/895.full.pdf.

25   Binzen, Carol A.; Swan, Pamela D.; Manore, Melinda M.; "Postexercise oxygen consumption and substrate use after resistance exercise in women." *Medicine & Science in Sports & Exercise.* June 2001. Volume 33—Issue 6, pages 932–938. Available at: http://journals.lww.com/acsm-msse/Abstract/2001/06000/Postexercise_oxygen_ consumption_and_substrate_use.12.aspx.

26   Boreham, C. A. G.; Kennedy, R. A.; Murphy M H; et al. "Training effects of short bouts of stair climbing on cardiorespiratory fitness, blood lipids, and homocysteine in sedentary young women." *British Journal of Sports Medicine,* January 2005. Volume 39—Issue 9. Available at: www.ncbi.nlm.nih.gov/pmc/articles/PMC1725304/pdf/v039p00590.pdf.

27   Author unknown. "Obesity in Children and Teens." Posted on the website for the American Academy of Child & Adolescent Psychiatry. May 28. Number 79. Available at: www.aacap.org/cs/root/facts_for_families/obesity_in_children_and_teens.

28   Semmler, Claudia; Ashcroft, Jo; van Jaarsveld, Cornelia H. M.; et al. "Development of overweight in children in relation to parental weight and socioeconomic status." *Obesity: A Research Journal.* Published online January 22, 2009. Available at: www .nature.com/oby/journal/v17/n4/full/oby2008621a.html.

29   Author unknown. "Obesity in Children and Teens." Posted on the website for the American Academy of Child & Adolescent Psychiatry. May 28. Number 79. Available at: www.aacap.org/cs/root/facts_for_families/obesity_in_children_and_teens.

30   Doolen, Jessica MSN, FNP; Alpert, Patricia T., DrPH, APN, FAANP; Miller, Sally, PhD, APN, FAANP. "Parental disconnect between perceived and actual weight status of children: a metasynthesis of the current research." *Journal of the American Academy of Nurse Practitioners,* March 2009. Volume 21—Issue 3. Pages 160–166. Available at: http://onlinelibrary.wiley.com/doi/10.1111/j.1745-7599.2008.00382.x/full.

31   Lowry, Kelly Walker, MS; Sallinen, Bethany J., PhD; Janicke, David M., PhD. "Self-Esteem in Pediatric Overweight Populations: Measurement of Self-Esteem." *Journal of Pediatric Psychology,* 2007. 32(10):1179–1195.

32   "Teasing about weight can affect pre-teens profoundly, study suggests." *ScienceDaily* September 24, 2010. Available at: www.sciencedaily.com/releases/2010/09/ 100907163521.htm. Referring to: Nelson, T. D.; and Steele, R. G. "Predictors of mental health practitioner use of evidence-based practices." *Administrative Policy in Mental Health and Mental Health Services Research,* July 2007. Volume 34—Number 4. Pages 319–330. Available at: www.ingentaconnect.com/content/klu/apih/2007/00000034/00 000004/00000111.

33   Smith, Stephen. "Taunting May Affect Health of Obese Youths." *The Boston Globe*, July 11, 2007. Available at: www.boston.com/yourlife/health/diseases/articles/2007/07/11/taunting_may_affect_health_of_obese_youths/. Referring to: Puhl, Rebecca M.; Latner, Janet D. "Stigma, obesity, and the health of the nation's children." *Psychological Bulletin,* July 2007. Volume 133—Issue 4, Pages 557–580.

34   Joseph Le; Zhang, Danna, MS; Menees, Spencer; et al. "'Vascular age' is advanced in children with atherosclerosis-promoting risk factors." *Circulation: Cardiovascular Imaging.* Published online before print, November 17, 2009. Available at: http://circimaging.ahajournals.org/content/3/1/8.full.

35   Feigin, Ralph D. *Textbook of Pediatric Infectious Diseases, Volume 1* (Elsevier Health Sciences, 2004). Page 674 et al.

36   Park, Steven Y., MD. *Sleep, Interrupted: A physician reveals the #1 reason why so many of us are sick and tired* (Jodev Press, LLC, 2008).

37   Website of the American Academy of Pediatrics. Portal for the "Prevention and Treatment of Childhood Overweight and Obesity." Available at: www.aap.org/health topics/overweight.cfm.

38   New Jersey Public Law 2007, c.45 (S1218) from Assembly bill No. 883 of the 212th State of New Jersey Legislature. Available at: www.njleg.state.nj.us/2006/Bills/A1000/883_I1.PDF.

39   Larson, Nicole I.; Neumark-Sztainer, Dianne; Hannan, Peter J.; et al. "Family meals during adolescence are associated with higher diet quality and healthful meal patterns during young adulthood." *Journal of the American Dietetic Association,* September 2007. Volume 107—Issue 9. Pages 1502–1510. Available at: www.adajournal.org/article/S0002-8223(07)01292-8/fulltext.

40   The National Center on Addiction and Substance Abuse at Columbia University (CASA). "National Survey of American Attitudes on Substance Abuse VIII: Teens and Parents." August 2003. Available at: www.casacolumbia.org/articlefiles/379-2003%20National%20Survey%20VIII.pdf.

41   Wing, Rena R.; Phelan, Suzanne. "Long-term weight loss maintenance." *American Journal of Clinical Nutrition*, July 2005. Volume 82, No. 1, Pages 222S–225S. Available at: www.ajcn.org/content/82/1/222S.long.

ABOUT THE AUTHORS

Bill Baroni graduated from the University of Virginia School of Law and George Washington University, where he majored in history, graduating magna cum laude with special honors. He was elected to the New Jersey State Senate in 2007 after serving two consecutive terms in the State Assembly. As a state senator, he served on the Health, Human Services, and Senior Citizens Committee; the Joint Committee on the Public Schools; and the Judiciary Committee, among many others. He also served on several boards for educational and nonprofit groups, including the New Jersey Symphony Orchestra and Visitation Home, an organization that builds homes for New Jerseyans with developmental disabilities. He is an Aspen-Rodel Fellow. Currently, he serves as deputy executive director of the Port Authority of New York and New Jersey. He also teaches education law, election law, and professional responsibility law at Seton Hall University Law School, where he was named Adjunct Professor of the Year in 2004 and 2011.

Damon DiMarco is the author of the oral histories *Tower Stories: An Oral History of 9/11* (with a foreword by Tom Kean, chairman of the Independent 9/11 Commission), and *Heart of War: Soldiers' Voices from Iraq*. He has also written books on acting: *The Actor's Art & Craft* with William Esper (featuring a foreword by Pulitzer Prize–winner David Mamet) and *The Quotable Actor: 1001 Pearls of Wisdom from Actors Talking about Acting*; and the collaborations *Out of Bounds: Coming Out of Sexual Abuse, Addiction, and My Life of Lies in the NFL Closet* with former offensive lineman Roy Simmons, and *My Two Chinas: The Memoir of a Chinese Counterrevolutionary* with Baiqiao Tang (featuring a foreword by His Holiness, the Dalai Lama). A professional actor as well as a writer, Damon has appeared in primetime and daytime television programs, commercials, independent films, regional theater, and trade shows. He has written for the stage, screen, and television, and taught acting on the faculties of Drew University in Madison, New Jersey, and the New York Film Academy in Manhattan.